Contents

Foreword   iv
About the author   vi
Acknowledgements   vii

Introduction   1

Part 1   An explanation of Models of Care   **5**
  1   Introducing Models of Care   7

Part 2   The patient's journey through Models of Care   **25**
  2   'I don't have a drug problem'   27
  3   Engaging with the drug service   41
  4   Alcohol and referral on for more support   53
  5   Counselling begins, preparing for the day programme   61
  6   Using on top, and a way ahead emerges   77
  7   Urging change, preparing for detoxification   93
  8   Treatment continues, preparing to move on   117
  9   Endings, suicide attempt and a new beginning?   135

Part 3   Reflecting on the success of Models of Care for this patient   **147**
  10   Reflections   149

Reflecting on Mark's journey through Models of Care: a psychiatrist's perspective   153

Reflecting on Mark's journey through Models of Care: a family therapy perspective   159

Emerging themes: reflections of a nurse consultant   163

Conclusion   167

References   173

Index   175

Foreword

Models of Care, commissioned by the Department of Health, is the best attempt to date to bring some order to the fairly dishevelled and idiosyncratic profession of treating people with drug problems. For over 50 years, drug treatment has grown up in a relatively experimental and organic way across the United Kingdom. There was little agreement as to what was the right way to carry out treatment and there was equal dissension about what was the wrong way. The result was that where you lived dictated the care you would receive: the classic 'postcode lottery'.

Treatment was often 'service-centred', or 'treatment-centred', as opposed to 'client-centred', offering what the service had always offered instead of tailoring the care to address the needs of the client. Despite the findings of research and mounting evidence, treatment services chose to implement the findings of studies that complemented their own philosophy and practice while ignoring the others that contradicted their care. As a drug user, if you fitted into the rules, regulations and philosophy of the agency you stumbled into, you were in luck. If you did not, there was the door. It is no wonder that services around the country had an average drop-out rate of 50%.

The mission of Models of Care was to change all that. Commissioned by the Department of Health, Models of Care was written by a large team of practitioners and academics, of which I was one. It took over a year to pull all the evidence together from the UK and internationally about what constitutes good treatment and care for drug misuse. Written in four chapters, Models of Care defines the treatment that everyone in the UK should expect and be entitled to receive to work with and help them overcome a drug problem.

Models of Care has been accepted and generally embraced by the drug treatment world. It has provided additional legitimacy to their work and a framework to work within. The Department of Health has endorsed the work and given it the status of National Service Framework for drug treatment. It is now the role of the National Treatment Agency on Substance Misuse (NTA) to oversee the implementation of Models of Care across the country.

There has been an 18-month implementation timetable for services, during which time those with the responsibility to organise services, such as Drug Action Teams (DATs), have to comply with the structural and systems improvements called for in Models of Care. But it will be years before all the aspects of Models of Care are fully in place in every part of the country. Change is not easy and, despite trying, Models of Care cannot provide answers to every situation. Local decisions still need to be made in implementing certain aspects of Models of Care.

Models of Care is a reference book. It is an encyclopaedia of what constitutes good care for drug treatment. But it is dry and difficult to digest. As one of the authors, I am at liberty to admit this fact.

That is what makes this book, *Models of Care for Drug Service Provision* by Richard Bryant-Jefferies, so fascinating and useful. It breathes life into a rather dull and abstract subject. Through the life of Mark, a fictitious drug user, and a range of professionals he comes into contact with over a three-month period, you get to experience drug treatment through the eyes of the service user.

It is not always a smooth ride in this process called treatment. It is full of bumps and U-turns along the way. The fictitious journey Mark takes rings true to my 20-plus years of working in this field and watching numerous clients, like Mark, start down this road.

Through all Mark's twists and turns, Models of Care is shown to be the route map that binds a lot of separate roads and paths into a system of care to help Mark, and people like Mark, come to terms with their drug use and take back control of their lives. Mark is no angel and, like most people, his problems are not always simple. Many steps along the road are painful and could so easily go wrong. There is a minefield of physical and emotional problems to manage and eventually overcome.

This new book is a wonderful reminder that we are dealing first and foremost with human beings who are complex, vulnerable and who also happen to have a drug problem. Our treatment professionals need to be well informed, up to date and responsive to the needs of clients like Mark. They also need to be understanding, tolerant and resourceful. Models of Care assists them by providing a framework within which to work and by helping to bind together the range of professionals and services into a system of care.

Don Lavoie
Performance Manager
National Treatment Agency
March 2004

About the author

Richard Bryant-Jefferies qualified as a person-centred counsellor/therapist in 1994 and remains passionate about the application and effectiveness of this approach. Between early 1995 and mid-2003, Richard worked at a community drug and alcohol service in Surrey, though more recently he has taken up a position managing NHS substance misuse services in the Royal Borough of Kensington and Chelsea in London, within the Central and North West London Mental Health NHS Trust. He has experience of offering both counselling and supervision in NHS, GP and private settings, and has provided training through 'alcohol awareness and response' workshops.

Richard had his first book on a counselling theme published in 2001, *Counselling the Person Beyond the Alcohol Problem* (Jessica Kingsley Publishers), providing theoretical yet practical insights into the application of the person-centred approach within the context of the 'cycle of change' model that has been widely adopted to describe the process of change in the field of addiction. Since then he has been writing for the *Living Therapy* series, producing an ongoing series of person-centred dialogues: *Problem Drinking*, *Time Limited Therapy in Primary Care*, *Counselling a Survivor of Child Sexual Abuse*, *Counselling a Recovering Drug User*, *Counselling Young People* and *Counselling for Progressive Disability*. The aim of the series is to bring the reader a direct experience of the counselling process, an exposure to the thoughts and feelings of both client and counsellor as they encounter each other on the therapeutic journey, and an insight into the value and importance of supervision.

Richard is keen to bring the experience of the therapeutic process, from the standpoint and application of the person-centred approach, to a wider audience. He is convinced that the principles and attitudinal values of this approach and the emphasis it places on the therapeutic relationship are key to helping people create greater authenticity both in themselves and in their lives, leading to a fuller and more satisfying human experience.

Acknowledgements

I would like to thank those who have contributed to this book: Jan Annan, who commented on the draft from her perspective as a member of the team that wrote *Models of Care*; and Dr William Shanahan, Consultant Psychiatrist, Kevin Simmons, Alison Smith, Francesca Trombaccia and Dennis Yandoli, Family Therapists, all working for the Substance Misuse Service within Central and North West London Mental Health NHS Trust. It has been important to widen the angle, so to speak, and to include perspectives from people working within other professions; professionals who have many years of experience of working within the substance misuse field and who know, from their own work with clients and with service development, what works and what does not, what is helpful and what hinders recovery.

I would also like to take this opportunity of acknowledging and thanking Movena Lucas who, by encouraging me to apply for my current job (which involved my preparing a presentation on Models of Care), triggered the chain of events that led to the writing of this book.

I am also grateful for the many discussions and conversations I have had with a variety of professionals regarding drug service provision over the years. My own experience of working in a community service – Acorn Community Drug and Alcohol Service in Surrey – has also been a factor in shaping my thoughts along with my current work as Sector Manager (Kensington and Chelsea), Substance Misuse Services, Central and North West London Mental Health NHS Trust.

We are indebted to the National Treatment Agency for allowing us to reproduce substantial portions of the Models of Care document in Chapter 1, all of which is in the public domain. This was essential to anchor the book to the current policies and strategies that aim to improve the quality of services and equity of access for all drug users.

Finally, to everyone at Radcliffe Publishing whose editorial skills have once again drawn together many threads to produce this book, and whose belief in the importance not only of the theme of this book, but also the style of presentation, has been so encouraging. Thank you once again.

Introduction

Drug problems affect us all, directly or indirectly. Perhaps a family member has or has had a drug problem. Maybe we have ourselves. Or it could be that we have been burgled by someone needing goods to sell on for a fix or two. But even if we have not been affected directly in this way, we are indirectly affected by the simple fact of our taxes being spent on drug treatment programmes, on the health and social care effects of drug use, and on criminal justice responses to illicit use. Drug use impacts on us all, to a greater or lesser extent.

Until the end of the last century, services were developed locally and there were huge amounts of competitive bidding for resources to develop services. Sometimes there was good co-operation between statutory and non-statutory services; in other areas bidding wars governed service provision. There might be little co-operation and communication between services. A culture of mistrust developed in some areas. Service provision varied from area to area. Good staff struggled to maintain quality service with increasing caseloads, and increasingly chaotic and demanding clients with new designer drugs being added to the already potent chemical cocktails from the past.

The National Treatment Agency (NTA) was established as 'a special health authority, created by the Government in 2001, with a remit to increase the availability, capacity and effectiveness of treatment for drug misuse in England' (NTA, 2002, p. 11) and has as its overall purpose the goal of 'doubling the number of people in effective, well-managed drug treatment from 100,000 in 1998 to 200,000 in 2008; and to increase the proportion of people completing or appropriately continuing treatment, year on year. This is in line with the UK drug strategy targets' (NTA, 2002, p. ii).

At the time of writing, drug and alcohol services are in the process of preparing for implementing the National Treatment Agency's 'Models of Care' system. This initiative will have a far-reaching effect on drug services throughout England. *Models of Care* has been published in two parts, both of which are available in hard copy (details at the back of this book) and online at www.nta.nhs.uk. The Models of Care system is composed of five elements: a four-tiered framework for drug and alcohol treatment services, integrated care pathways, assessment within a tiered system, care planning and care co-ordination, and monitoring. We will describe these in more detail in Chapter 1.

Without doubt, the way Models of Care is implemented will vary greatly across the country, and the fact that each Drug Action Team (DAT) area has in effect been left to formulate its own process means there is a lot of opportunity for services to collaborate on systems that will have relevance to a particular geographical area, offering scope for different areas of emphasis and service provision reflecting client need.

In writing this book I hope to contribute not only to the process of implementation, but also to stimulate thought and discussion around what it means to provide more 'client-' rather than 'treatment-centred' drug services. I believe we have to move away from any notion of 'one-size-fits-all' or, rather, one treatment response as being the answer to every drug user's difficulties. Models of Care should help ensure a range of treatment responses are available to all people regardless of where they live. Without doubt, assessment and care co-ordination are going to require appropriately trained individuals in order to ensure that the integrated set of care pathways that are formulated for a given service user will be genuinely tailored to meet that person's needs.

This book has been written to present a fictitious account of a client with a drug problem engaging with services as they might exist under the Models of Care system. It includes comment boxes on the process, on technical aspects of treatment and around issues that can arise in the treatment process. In places, these boxes also include references to the Models of Care system, highlighting what is being offered within the narrative and how it equates to levels of assessment or tiered treatment interventions. The book also includes three sections from leading professionals in the field, commenting on the account and on their professional view of Models of Care. I hope that the varied styles of the writers and the format in this book will serve to appeal widely, to all who will find themselves working either within, or in collaboration with, services within the Models of Care system.

Bringing together what is at times a technical and informative style with a more narrative 'story' has been a challenge. Telling a story in the context of a defined system of practice which has not yet actually been established is also an interesting process. Of course, there are many other treatment modalities that might have been included within the text of this book, and a range of other professionals that will be providing care pathways for clients with substance misuse problems. The text keeps to a health/medical and therapeutic emphasis in order to demonstrate their application. However, the range of professionals and services that might have been involved in the unfolding scenario could have been wider, and this will be reflected on further towards the end of the book.

A colloquial style is used within the narrative, seeking to reflect the language of the real world rather than that of the textbook. However, the language and style that individuals adopt will differ and so there is no intention here to represent a kind of stereotypical style of working or some kind of archetypal characterisation.

Models of Care for Drug Service Provision attempts to appeal to a wide audience, but perhaps those for whom it will have most appeal will be those who know little or nothing of drug service provision, those working within treatment modalities outside of those described in this book who want an insight into specific areas of Tier 3 treatment provision, and counsellors who wish to broaden their understanding of working with drug-using clients. For the specialist I hope that it will offer 'a good read', and an opportunity to reflect on their own practice and deepen their understanding of how this fits into the Models of Care system. It will also have relevance for clients, and for relatives and carers of clients, who may wish to deepen their understanding of drug service provision. In using the narrative approach I have sought to bring the experience alive, to draw response and reaction from the reader.

Have I described an 'ideal client'? Perhaps. In reality there could be more problems arising and the process may well have been more drawn out. Many clients do not complete treatment, returning to old patterns of use sometimes, or moving out of area. Clients can take a lot longer to engage with, sometimes. Not everyone engages so quickly with the motivation that the client, Mark, achieves. So I hope this will be taken into account. Also, I am not trying to describe a 'right way' of working with clients, but 'a way' which I hope not only encourages greater understanding of Models of Care but also thoughts and reflection on what services are offering and how they can better collaborate in the interest of the client's health and well-being.

PART I

An explanation of Models of Care

CHAPTER 1

Introducing Models of Care

The following chapter is very much drawn from section 2 of the NTA's *Models of Care* publication (2002). Rather than attempt to rewrite what has already been said, and perhaps lose some of the definition in the process, it seemed more sensible to collate key ideas and present them in a somewhat compressed and hopefully readable form.

> The *Models of Care* document overall sets out a national framework for the commissioning of adult treatment for drug misuse (drug treatment) expected to be available in every part of England to meet the needs of diverse local populations. (NTA, 2002, p. 3)

This is a major step forward, establishing a national and co-ordinated approach to drug treatment.

> The overriding concept behind Models of Care is that Drug Action Teams (DATs) should be seeking to develop an integrated drug treatment system in their area, not just a series of separate services. In the last few years, DAT members have received increasing funding to expand the capacity of the various modalities of treatment, but it is also felt that efforts must be made to combine these modalities into a seamless system of 'care pathways' for patients. The Models of Care approach describes how these processes of care would work, based on the menu of treatment services that have already been incorporated into DAT treatment plans, but now expressed in terms of 4 treatment 'tiers'. (NTA, 2002, p. 5)

Implementation targets

The NTA has set certain implementation targets before the DATs:

> To have agreed by *January 2003* the joint planning mechanism, and lead individual, that will be responsible in a DAT area for pursing the implementation of *Models of Care*. By *October 2003* to have completed an assessment of whether the assessment and referral mechanisms (and treatment providers) in your DAT area are operating according to the evidence-based patient placement

criteria and treatment protocols outlined in the *Models of Care* document. The next step, due by *November 2003*, is to agree and publish a local referral, screening and triage system, supported by an information-sharing policy, making clear the referral points into the drug treatment system, who is responsible for conducting the various levels of assessment, how referrals are made into the main modalities of treatment, the protocols for information sharing and exchange, and the assessment forms and instruments that will be used. Finally, by *March 2004* locally defined care pathways, and a local system of care co-ordination should have been agreed and published. (NTA, 2002, p. 8)

A look at the NTA website will give you updates and information on the developments taking place around the country. Integrated care pathways are being generated, for instance, defining the responses to a diagnosed dual diagnosis, or to specific aspects of drug treatment needs, for instance, injectable prescribing.

Assessment forms are also being generated for use across DAT regions, ensuring that agencies are working to similar criteria and that information exchange can occur between agencies, and between tiers.

Four tiers

These are described as follows.

- Tier 1: Non-substance misuse specific services requiring interface with drug and alcohol treatment.
- Tier 2: Open access drug and alcohol treatment services.
- Tier 3: Structured community-based drug treatment services.
- Tier 4 services: Residential services for drug and alcohol misusers:
  – Tier 4a: Residential drug and alcohol misuse specific services
  – Tier 4b: Highly specialist non-substance misuse specific services.

Tier 1: Non-substance misuse specific services requiring interface with drug and alcohol treatment

Tier 1 services do not have a substance-specific role, but they provide an opportunity for screening drug misusers, engaging with them and initiating referral on to local drug and alcohol treatment services in Tiers 2 and 3. Tier 1 provision for drug and alcohol misusers may also include assessment, services to reduce drug-related harm, and liaison or joint working with Tiers 2 and 3 specialist drug and alcohol treatment services. Tier 1 services are crucial to providing services in conjunction with more specialised drug and alcohol services (e.g. general medical care for drug misusers in community-based or residential substance misuse treatment or housing support and aftercare for drug misusers leaving residential care or prison).

Tier 1 services are offered by a wide range of professionals, including primary care or general medical services, general social workers, teachers, community pharmacists, probation officers, housing officers and homeless persons' units. These professionals are not substance misuse specialists, but will have been trained to recognise and assess the presence of drug and alcohol misuse in order to refer people on to other agencies offering specific treatment responses.

The importance of training is emphasised in Models of Care, to ensure that professionals working in Tier 1 services can effectively identify and assess drug misuse. It is likely that there will be a need for developing liaison posts so that Tier 2 and 3 services can collaborate with Tier 1, for instance in areas where there are high levels of pregnancy and maternal health need, or a high transient homeless population attracted into the area by the presence of hostel accommodation.

Models of Care emphasises that:

Drug misusers in all DATs in England must have access at local levels to the following Tier 1 services located within local general health and social care services:

- a full range of healthcare (primary, secondary and tertiary), social care, housing, vocational and other services
- drug and alcohol screening, assessment and referral mechanisms to drug treatment services from generic, health, social care, housing and criminal justice services
- the management of drug misusers in generic health, social care and criminal justice settings (e.g. police custody)
- health promotion advice and information
- hepatitis B vaccination programmes for drug misusers and their families. (NTA, 2002, p. 17)

Tier 2: Open access drug and alcohol treatment services

Tier 2 services will offer a range of services for drug misusers, including needle exchange, drug (and alcohol) advice and information services, and general support, including harm reduction support, not delivered in the context of a care plan, and low-threshold prescribing programmes aimed at engaging opioid misusers with limited motivation, while offering an opportunity to undertake motivational work and reduce drug-related harm. Specialist substance misuse social workers can provide services within this tier, including the provision of access to social work advice, childcare/parenting assessment, and assessment of social care needs. Shared-care services with primary healthcare are also included in this tier, though this may vary depending upon the complexity of the clients' needs who are being supported through this approach.

A key element in defining the services within this tier is their low threshold of access, and the limited requirements on clients to receive services. Access will be by self-referral as well as via other agencies: Tier 1 who have identified a problem requiring Tier 2 intervention or triage assessment that may be carried out by local Tier 2 services, or higher Tier 3 or 4 services when a client has been assessed as requiring the kind of community support and intervention of a Tier 2 service as part of a care planned and care co-ordinated response.

The aim of the treatment in Tier 2 is to engage drug and alcohol misusers in drug treatment and reduce drug-related harm. Tier 2 services do not necessarily require a high level of commitment to structured programmes or a complex or lengthy assessment process. Models of Care points out that Tier 2 services require competent drug and alcohol specialist workers, and that the tiers do not imply lower skills within lower tiers.

> Drug misusers in all DATs in England must have access to the following Tier 2 open-access specialist drug interventions within their local area:
>
> - drug- and alcohol-related advice, information and referral services for misusers (and their families), including easy access or drop-in facilities
> - services to reduce risks caused by injecting drug misuse, including needle exchange facilities (in drug treatment services and pharmacy-based schemes)
> - other services that minimise the spread of blood-borne diseases to drug misusers, including service-based and outreach facilities
> - services that minimise the risk of overdose and other drug- and alcohol-related harm
> - outreach services (detached; peripatetic and domiciliary) targeting high-risk and local priority groups
> - specialist drug and alcohol screening and assessment, care planning and management
> - criminal justice screening, assessment and referral services (e.g. arrest referral, CARATS [Counselling, Assessment, Referral, Advice and Through-care Services])
> - motivational and brief interventions for drug and alcohol service users
> - community-based low-threshold prescribing services.
> (NTA, 2002, pp. 17–18)

Tier 3: Structured community-based drug treatment services

Tier 3 structured services include psychotherapeutic interventions and structured counselling, as well as motivational interventions, methadone maintenance programmes, community detoxification, and day care provided either as a drug- and alcohol-free programme or as an adjunct to methadone treatment. Community-based aftercare programmes for drug and alcohol misusers leaving residential rehabilitation or prison are also included in Tier 3 services. Such services are likely to be required to work closely with other specialist services to meet the needs of specific client groups. For example, where the drug users have a psychiatric co-morbidity there will be a need for substance misuse and mental health services to work closely together.

Tier 3 services require that the drug and alcohol misusers receive a comprehensive assessment and have a care plan which is agreed with the client, generally including a structured programme of care which places certain requirements on attendance and behaviour, and commitment from both parties: the service provider and the client. Models of Care stresses the importance of a care co-ordinator for those clients 'whose needs cross several domains . . . responsible for co-ordination of that individual's care on behalf of all the agencies and services involved' (NTA, 2002, p. 18). Any changes to a care plan must follow consultation with the drug and alcohol misuser.

Drug misusers in all DATs in England must have access to the following Tier 3 structured drug treatment services normally provided within their local area and occasionally by neighbouring DAT or regionally located facilities:

- specific community care assessment and care management
- new care co-ordination services for drug misusers with complex needs (provided by suitably trained practitioners)
- specialist structured community-based detoxification services
- a range of specialist structured community-based stabilisation and maintenance prescribing services
- shared-care prescribing and support treatment via primary care
- a range of structured, care planned counselling and therapies
- community-based Drug Treatment and Testing Order drug treatment
- structured day programmes (in urban and semi-urban areas)
- other structured community-based drug misuse services targeting specific groups (e.g. stimulant misusers, young people in transition to adulthood, black and minority ethnic groups, women drug misusers, drug misusing offenders, those with HIV and AIDS, drug misusers with psychiatric problems)
- liaison drug misuse services for acute medical and psychiatric sectors (e.g. pregnancy, mental health)
- liaison drug misuse services for local social services and social care sectors (e.g. child protection, housing and homelessness, family services)
- throughcare and aftercare programmes or support. (NTA, 2002, p. 19)

Tier 4 services: Residential services for drug and alcohol misusers

Tier 4a: Residential drug and alcohol misuse specific services

Tier 4a services are aimed at individuals with a high level of presenting need. Services in this tier include: inpatient drug and alcohol detoxification or stabilisation services; drug and alcohol residential rehabilitation units; and residential drug crisis intervention centres. Clients require a care co-ordinator prior to accessing services at this tier and it is recognised that a high level of commitment will be required from the client, along with a certain degree of preparatory work (except in crisis situations when this may not be possible). Generally access to Tier 4a services will be from lower tiers or via community care assessment.

Tier 4b: Highly specialist non-substance misuse specific services

Tier 4b services include specialist liver units and forensic services for mentally ill offenders. Some highly specialist Tier 4b services also provide specialist liaison services to Tiers 1–4a services (e.g. specialist hepatitis nurses, HIV liaison clinics, genito-urinary medicine).

> Drug misusers in all DATs in England must have access to the following Tier 4 services, most likely provided at a multi-DAT or regional or national level:

- specialist drug and alcohol residential rehabilitation programmes (including a range of 12-step, faith-based, and eclectic programmes)
- generic and drug specialist semi-structured residential care (e.g. half-way houses, semi-supported accommodation)
- specialist Drug Treatment and Testing Order treatment (residential options)
- inpatient drug misuse treatment, ideally provided by specialist drug misuse units, or alternatively by designated beds in generic (mental) health services
- highly specialist forms of residential rehabilitation units or other residential services (inpatient, prison) with a drug misuse treatment component (e.g. women and children, crisis intervention, dual diagnosis)
- relevant Tier 4b services, including HIV or liver disease units, vein clinics, residential services for young people, and so forth. (NTA, 2002, p. 20)

Integrated care pathways

An integrated care pathway (ICP) is essentially a description of the nature and anticipated course of treatment for a particular client and a predetermined plan of treatment. Each treatment modality within the tier system will be clearly defined so that a client, referred for a particular treatment response, will be clear as to what they are receiving.

ICPs are important for drug and alcohol misusers for the following reasons:

- Drug and alcohol misusers often have multiple problems which require effective co-ordination of treatment.
- Several specialist and generic service providers may be involved in the care of a drug and alcohol misuser simultaneously or consecutively.
- A drug and alcohol misuser may have continuing and evolving care needs requiring referral to different tiers of service over time.

- ICPs ensure consistency and parity of approach nationally (i.e. a drug misuser accessing a particular treatment modality should receive the same response wherever they access care).
- ICPs ensure that access to care is not based on individual clinical decisions or historical arrangements. (NTA, 2002, p. 26)

Services are developing flow charts to describe ICPs for specific diagnoses which, while an important structure, nevertheless may need to be adjusted for the specific needs of individual clients, and will certainly have highlighted areas of specific relevance to an individual client, for instance, the client with a history of disengaging from services may require a more comprehensive strategy for responding to this problem area.

Models of Care stresses:

Integrated care pathways should have the following elements:

- a definition of the treatment modality provided
- aims and objectives of the treatment modality
- definition of the client group served
- eligibility criteria (including priority groups)
- exclusions criteria or contraindications
- referral pathway
- screening and assessment processes
- development of agreed treatment goals
- description of the treatment process or phases
- care co-ordination
- departure planning, aftercare and support
- onward referral pathways
- services with which the modality interfaces. (NTA, 2002, pp. 26–7)

ICPs need to be comprehensive in order to ensure that the treatment planned includes all the necessary elements required by a particular drug or alcohol misuser. Therefore an important aspect of the Models of Care system is assessment.

Assessment

Within the complex world of drug and alcohol misuse, the need for highly skilled assessment is vital to ensure that a client's needs are identified and that they are matched with services that provide the appropriate treatment response(s). Drug use becomes ingrained over years. Early identification of problems is to be encouraged so that treatment can be offered at the earliest opportunity.

Three levels of assessment will be provided from within the tiers as follows:

- Level 1: Screening and referral assessment (Tiers 1 and 4b)
- Level 2: Drug and alcohol misuse triage assessment (Tiers 2, 3 and 4)

- Level 3: Comprehensive drug and alcohol misuse assessment (Tiers 3 and 4a and some Tier 2). (NTA, 2002, p. 29)

The Drug and Alcohol National Occupational Standards (DANOS) outline the basic competencies that are required by professionals for the different levels of screening and assessment of clients who present with drug and alcohol problems (Skills for Health, 2002).

The aim should be for all personnel in Tiers 1 and 4b services to have basic training in the identification of drug misuse problems and to be familiar with local drug service provision for referral on and/or liaison.

Level 1 assessment: Initial screening

Level 1 assessment is less complex than Levels 2 or 3, but at a minimum it needs to include the following:

- identification of a drug or alcohol misuse problem
- identification of related or co-existent problems (e.g. physical, psychological, social)
- identification of immediate risks (e.g. self-harm, harm to others, physical and/or mental health emergencies)
- an assessment of the urgency of referral. (NTA, 2002, p. 32)

The outcome of Level 1 assessment will be referral of the drug or alcohol misuser, with the appropriate degree of urgency, to the appropriate service. This may be to a drug service, but it could be to a non-substance service where the immediate need is, for instance, suicide, parasuicide, overdose, child protection. There will be occasions when referral to both will be necessary so that a client is already known and can be offered assessment by the drug agency after the crisis has been addressed.

Models of Care indicates that:

The Level 1 screening assessment tool and Level 2 triage assessment need to have the following characteristics:

- It needs to be agreed locally and adapted to meet local needs and local service provision.
- It must achieve referrals against agreed criteria.
- It must be categorical, concise, comprehensive and straightforward to apply.
- It can be audited against locally agreed standards. (NTA, 2002, p. 32)

Feedback from the services in receipt of referral should be made to the referring services, to inform the referral process.

Level 2: Drug misuse triage assessment

Level 2 assessment should be carried out by trained individuals within all drug treatment services (Tiers 2–4a). The assessment will build on what has been recognised within the initial screening (where the referral has been initiated by a Tier 1 service). It should be undertaken to agreed criteria and to a standardised format across the local area. Models of Care suggests that 'information obtained in a Level 2 assessment should be appropriately shared with all agencies to which the drug and alcohol misuser is subsequently referred', highlighting the importance of this in relation to 'identified risks and risk management' (NTA, 2002, p. 32). Models of Care also places high emphasis on risk assessment to a locally agreed protocol and using standardised documentation across all drug and alcohol treatment services, to include: risks to the individual drug and alcohol misuser (e.g. self-harm, self-neglect, exploitation), risks to others (e.g. homicide, child protection issues, violence), historical risk factors disclosed (e.g. past history of self-harm, history of disengagement from services), presenting risk factors (e.g. threats to kill, suicidal ideas), and drug overdose and other drug-related harm.

Triage assessment is likely to be a client's first face-to-face contact with a drug treatment agency, and therefore this level of assessment should be available within all drug and alcohol services and community care assessment teams. Clients are referred on for treatment in accordance with locally agreed criteria; the aim is to ensure that clients receive the treatment most appropriate to their need, and 'to ensure that staff carrying out Level 2 assessments are not tempted to keep hold of clients in order to meet performance targets or because of beliefs that their own approaches are best' (NTA, 2002, p. 33). Triage assessment comprises a more in-depth assessment of the person's drug and alcohol problem including the complexity of the presenting need and the client's willingness to engage with services, identification of the services required, the level of risk, and the degree of urgency.

Level 2 triage assessment is not intended to be a comprehensive assessment. The aims of Level 2 assessment are to:

- identify and respond to emergency or acute problems
- identify risks to the substance misuser or others (through risk assessment)
- ensure appropriate referral based on the level of expertise and intensity of the intervention required
- ensure common processes and criteria across a range of local drug (and alcohol) treatment services for professionals undertaking triage assessment
- route drug and alcohol misusers with more complex needs into a care co-ordinated programme of care, including comprehensive drug and alcohol misuse assessment
- allow individuals with less complex needs to access less complex and/or less structured drug services (e.g. advice services, harm reduction services).

Level 2 assessment needs to include the following:

- risk assessment: identification of immediate risks (e.g. self-harm, harm to others, physical and/or mental health emergencies)
- an assessment of the urgency of referral
- brief assessment of drug and alcohol misuse problem
- brief assessment of client readiness to engage in types of treatment
- assessment of whether or not the client meets the criteria for needing more comprehensive (Level 3) assessment and care co-ordination.

We recommend that only named (or approved) staff with the appropriate skills, training and competence should undertake Level 2 assessment of drug and alcohol misusers. Staff undertaking Level 2 assessment must have had special training which includes:

- standardised training on how to interpret guidelines and criteria and also how to apply them
- learning about the expertise and skills of professionals in the various treatment modalities (training sessions carried out by staff in the different modalities)
- risk assessment and risk management
- basic drug and alcohol misuse assessment skills. (NTA, 2002, pp. 33–4)

By way of explanation, Models of Care continues: 'The purpose of the Level 2 assessment process is therefore to gather information to identify need and guide the client to appropriate services, and also to maximise the likelihood of client engagement in treatment' (NTA, 2002, p. 35).

Assessors at Tier 2 will need to have received the appropriate level of training to ensure that they have an appreciation and understanding, and the necessary skills, to encourage clients to convey the information needed upon which their assessment will be based. How problematic is a client's drug use? Is it generating dependence and risk of withdrawal? Does the client need assessment for substitute prescribing or full assessment for possible mental health problems? Does the client need a physical check-up from a clinical nurse specialist? Are there physical symptoms being described that could be linked to drug use? Does the client need to be seen by a doctor and, if so, how urgently? It will be vital that Tier 2 services are able to distinguish those clients suited to their package of interventions, and those that need a more comprehensive assessment of their needs.

Level 3: Comprehensive substance misuse assessment

Models of Care recognises that comprehensive assessment is an ongoing process, not a one-off event. It will be carried out by staff working at Tiers 3 and 4, and in some instances at Tier 2.

The Level 3 comprehensive assessment tool should have the following characteristics:

- It needs to be agreed locally and adapted to meet local needs and local ser-
  vice provision.
- It must achieve outcomes against agreed criteria.
- It must be comprehensive and inclusive.
- It must provide clear conclusions and form the basis of a clear care plan.
- It can be audited against locally agreed standards.

Level 3 assessments should be targeted at drug and alcohol misusers with more
complex needs and/or at those who require more complex and/or structured
care programmes. The criteria for comprehensive assessments are identical to
the criteria for care co-ordination, namely drug and/or alcohol misusers who
present with one or more of the following:

- significant drug and alcohol misuse problems in two or more problem
  domains
- in need of structured and/or intensive intervention
- significant psychiatric and/or physical co-morbidity
- significant risk of harm to self or others
- in contact with multiple service providers
- pregnancy or children 'at risk'
- history of disengagement from drug treatment services. (NTA, 2002, p. 35)

So, clearly Level 3 assessment will not be for everyone. Indeed, as one progresses
through the tiers it is likely that the greater number of clients with drug problems
will be accessing services from the lower tiers; only those with much more complex conditions arising out of, or linked with, their drug use will reach Tier 3.
Comprehensive assessment:

should, at a minimum, allow assessment of the following domains:

- drug use (including type of drug(s), quantity/frequency of use, pattern of
  use, route of administration, source of drug)
- alcohol use (including quantity/frequency of use, pattern of use, whether
  above 'safe' level, alcohol dependence symptoms)
- psychological problems (including self-harm, history of abuse/trauma,
  depression, severe psychiatric co-morbidity, contact with mental health
  services)
- physical problems (including complications of drug/alcohol use, pregnancy, blood-borne infections/risk behaviours, liver disease, abscesses,
  overdose, enduring or severe physical disabilities)
- social issues (including childcare issues, partners, domestic violence,
  family, housing, employment, benefits, financial problems)
- legal problems (including arrests, fines, outstanding charges/warrants,
  probation, imprisonment, violent offences, criminal activity). (NTA, 2002,
  pp. 35–6)

Following assessment at Tier 3, clients will be allocated a care co-ordinator who will oversee and co-ordinate the care planning and treatment responses that have been agreed with the client.

Without doubt, the assessment process will need to be carried out by trained and competent people who have a clear understanding of the breadth and depth of the impact of problematic drug use. Clear assessment mechanisms will need to be established so that services can work towards similar standards and criteria for assessment. Standardised assessment forms will ease collaboration particularly if the components of the triage assessment are easily integrated into the comprehensive assessment process. One thing that irritates clients is the constant repetition through endless chains of assessment. There will also be a need for clearly integrated assessment mechanisms between drug and mental health services.

Of course, some services will have a leaning towards a particular area of care and concern: a social worker may be more oriented towards assessing social rather than healthcare needs, and health workers perhaps less oriented towards social care needs, hence the importance of multidisciplinary working and a readiness to refer on to other specialists to assess that which has been identified as an area of need but which may be beyond the competence of a particular professional. What must be guarded against is professional difference becoming a barrier to holistic assessment.

Assessment is an ongoing process and it will be important for clients to not only move up the tiers to services providing, for instance, specialist medical interventions, but also to move down as they stabilise, move on, and perhaps reduce the complexity of their needs. A threat to the effectiveness of the Models of Care system will come as a result of services inappropriately holding on to clients who, according to need, should be referred on. One reason why this can occur is where a service needs clients to maintain activity levels to justify funding. This has to be watched out for with external monitoring and evaluation where it is deemed that internal processes are not reflecting accurately what is occurring. There is also the case that clients may be held on to, particularly where the work has been long term and a familiar relationship has developed between a drug worker and a client, and/or there are unclear and unmonitored discharge policies. In healthcare settings, stabilised clients will need to be referred to other forms of support to free up specialists to work with those clients who are presenting in more complex and chaotic states. Again and again we come back to the importance of collaboration if the Models of Care system is to work.

Care planning and care co-ordination

Models of Care defines a care plan as:

> a structured, often multidisciplinary, and task-oriented individual care pathway plan, which details the essential steps in the care of a drug and alcohol

misuser and describes the drug and alcohol misuser's expected treatment and care course … [it] involves the translation of the needs, strength and risks identified by the assessment into a service response. It is used as a tool to monitor any changes in the situation of the drug and alcohol misuser and to keep other relevant professionals aware of these changes. (NTA, 2002, pp. 39–40)

Care planning and co-ordination seek to ensure that clients have access to services across the tiers and that service provision is followed through without unnecessary duplication or clients falling between services.

Good systems of care planning and care co-ordination will ensure that services are client-centred and not determined by the modalities provided by a particular agency. Such systems are intended to facilitate access to a programme of integrated and co-ordinated health and social care and to maximise client retention and minimise disengagement ('drop out') from the drug and alcohol treatment system.

The overarching principle of care planning and care co-ordination is that those who enter into structured drug and alcohol treatment services receive a written care plan which is agreed with the client and subject to regular review with the key worker or care co-ordinator. Drug and alcohol misusers who meet the criteria for care co-ordination should have access to a named person who acts as the care co-ordinator, to ensure that the care provided by different services is co-ordinated by one person to provide a comprehensive and integrated approach. (NTA, 2002, p. 39)

The care plan should be reviewed regularly in terms of its relevance, effectiveness and outcomes, unmet need, and client satisfaction with what is being provided. It should achieve the following:

- set the goals of treatment and milestones to be achieved (taking into account the views and treatment goals of the drug and alcohol misuser, and developed with their active participation)
- indicate the interventions planned and which agency and professional is responsible for carrying out the interventions
- make explicit reference to risk management and identify the risk management plan and contingency plans
- identify information sharing (what information will be given to other professionals/agencies, and under what circumstances)
- identify the engagement plan to be adopted with drug and alcohol misusers who are difficult to engage in the treatment system
- identify the review date (the date of the next review meeting is set and recorded at each meeting)
- reflect the cultural and ethnic background of the drug and alcohol misuser, as well as their gender and sexuality. (NTA, 2002, p. 40)

Two levels of care co-ordination are defined:

- Standard Care Co-ordination (equivalent to Standard Care Programme Approach [SCPA])
- Enhanced Care Co-ordination (equivalent to Enhanced Care Programme Approach [ECPA]). (NTA, 2002, pp. 40–1)

The criteria for care co-ordination are identical to the criteria for comprehensive assessment (NTA, 2002, p. 42).

Under enhanced care co-ordination and CPA [the Care Programme Approach], the expectation is that the client has severe mental health co-morbidity (e.g. schizophrenia, bipolar affective disorder, severe depression) and is thus subject to the national guidelines for enhanced CPA (NTA, 2002, p. 42). In such cases the client will generally be under the care of the Community Mental Health Team who take the lead in care co-ordination, with the drug and alcohol service taking responsibility for specific areas of the care plan, in line with the Department of Health guidance on dual diagnosis (*see* Department of Health, 2002).

> Enhanced CPA currently applies to those clients with severe mental health problems resulting in chronic disability or those clients who:
>
> - need a high level of support generally from more than one professional or agency
> - are subject to Section 117(2) of the Mental Health Act or Supervised Discharge under Section 25(a)
> - are on the Supervision Register. (NTA, 2002, p. 43)

With regard to clients on Drug Treatment and Testing Orders, Models of Care highlights the need for integration between care and sentence planning, with regular reviews and monitoring, and with neither service (probation or drug treatment) taking major decisions without mutual consultation.

Concerning the role of care co-ordinator, Models of Care says the following:

> The role of a care co-ordinator may involve the following responsibilities, depending on the locally agreed system:
>
> - to develop, manage and review documented care plans based on ongoing assessment (including risk assessment)
> - to ensure that the care plan takes account of the service user's presenting needs, and their culture, ethnicity, gender and sexuality
> - to carry out ongoing risk assessment and co-ordinate an appropriate risk management plan
> - to work towards engaging and retaining the drug (and alcohol) misuser in the treatment and care system
> - to co-ordinate care across the range of health and social care agencies
> - to act as a facilitator to help the service user to access other appropriate services

- to generate referrals
- to advise other professionals involved in the care of the service user of changes in the circumstances of the service user which may require a review or change of the care plan
- to ensure essential and appropriate information is shared between agencies
- to develop contingency and crisis management plans for service users with complex needs, where required
- to keep in touch with the service user
- to carry out an early follow-up of discharged service users
- to aim to re-engage service users who have dropped out of the drug treatment system. (NTA, 2002, pp. 43–4)

Emphasis is also placed on the competencies of the care co-ordinator, as outlined in the DANOS standards. These are the following:

- an understanding of drug and alcohol misuse
- comprehensive assessment skills, using locally agreed tools and protocols
- care co-ordination skills
- knowledge of local drug and alcohol treatment services and other relevant services and their respective roles
- knowledge of drug and alcohol misuse (including opiate, stimulant and polydrug misuse)
- competence in working with diversity, including awareness of race, culture and gender issues
- competence in the delivery of care to drug and alcohol misusers (including an understanding of substance misuse treatment and care)
- an understanding of the principles of and local policies on client confidentiality and appropriate sharing of information (including child protection in line with local Area Child Protection Committee [ACPC] guidelines). (NTA, 2002, p. 44)

In practice, care co-ordinators will probably be experienced members of a team or service. Only some staff will be competent to undertake this. Those with a care co-ordinator role are likely to need to have a smaller caseload than others. Care co-ordination is likely to include both extensive and intensive work with some individuals, and a lot of involvement liaising with other services.

Monitoring

There is an increasing imperative to monitor the activity, cost and outcomes of drug and alcohol treatment services. This reflects a desire to gauge the return on local and national investment and to ensure that resources are directed to effective treatment. (NTA, 2002, p. 46)

The monitoring of outcomes ensures that treatments offered are evaluated in their effectiveness and that clients receive the most effective treatments for their difficulties. A particularly important element of monitoring is ensuring systems for feedback from service users, again to inform the ongoing commissioning of services and to build increasing understanding, from practice, of what is effective. Models of Care draws attention to how:

> Clinical governance frameworks in the NHS and Best Value frameworks in local authorities are also frameworks of accountability to ensure that organisations are continuously improving the quality of their services and safeguarding high standards of care. In drug and alcohol treatment services, Quality in Alcohol and Drug Services (QuADS) standards on organisational management include specific standards on monitoring service activity and client outcome. Existing commissioning standards for those responsible for drug and alcohol treatment (Substance Misuse Advisory Service, 1999) includes explicit standards on contract monitoring and information gathering vis-à-vis local population needs. Commissioners have a critical role to play in developing local systems for monitoring activity and outcome. (NTA, 2002, p. 47)

Added to this, the NTA:

> is currently developing an informational strategy and minimum data set to support the implementation of Models of Care. The data set will be published as an addendum to Models of Care. The NTA data set will describe care received by the service user during each period of care and will be person-centred. It will also record outcome achieved through the treatment process. It is intended that the primary function of this data set will be to determine whether desired outcomes are achieved by drug treatment services. It is also intended that the data set will provide managers, clinicians and other professionals with better-quality information for clinical audit, service planning, management and contract monitoring. (NTA, 2002, p. 46)

Further elements of Models of Care

This introduction by no means describes every facet of the Models of Care system, simply the four-tier framework, assessment, integrated care pathways, care co-ordination and planning, and monitoring. Within the Models of Care document is further information that deals more specifically with treatment modalities, special groups and cross-cutting issues:

- information regarding specific drug misuse treatment modalities (advice and information, needle exchange facilities, care-planned counselling, structured day programmes, community prescribing, inpatient substance misuse treatment, residential rehabilitation)
- special groups (stimulant users, women drug users, black and minority ethnic populations, young people and substance misuse, substance-misusing parents, alcohol and alcohol misuse in drug misusers)

- cross-cutting issues (overdose, blood-borne diseases, psychiatric co-morbidity (dual diagnosis), outreach work, criminal justice, users, carers and self-help groups, complementary therapies, performance and outcome monitoring).

Young people

While this book is not designed to directly address the issues of working with young people with drug problems, it is important to be aware that young people have their own tiered system as follows.

- Tier 1: Services for all young people – education, information, early identification and screening.
- Tier 2: Services for vulnerable young people – harm reduction, reintegration, maintenance in mainstream services.
- Tier 3: Services for young problem substance misusers – focus on complex needs.
- Tier 4: Drug treatment services offering intensive interventions including prescribing, detoxification and residential treatment services. (Health Advisory Service, 1996)

Conclusion

What is important to stress is that Models of Care is a *system*, that while it has structure its effectiveness will be demonstrated through information flow and the relational factors that ensure good inter-agency co-operation and collaboration. Clients will need to flow through the system. Anything that obstructs this flow will need to be addressed.

Assessors at any level will need to be competent and, where necessary, training will be required. The importance of the quality of assessment cannot be over-emphasised. However, assessment must take into account the client's perspective and, where possible, carer perspectives and experiences as well. How does the client view their drug use? Does this match the carer's view? What concerns are present for drug user and carer? What help is seen to be needed by the parties involved? Where there are clear differences between a client, a carer or carers and the assessor and/or the care co-ordinator, how might they be resolved satisfactorily? Powerful familial and relational dynamics can be, and often are, present where drug use is involved.

Care co-ordinators, in particular, will need to receive appropriate levels of support and supervision (personal and professional) to ensure that they can stand clear of some of the powerful dynamics in order to maintain clarity. But at times this may be lost and supervision should offer a learning opportunity to understand process and to reformulate responses to clients and carers. It will also be important for care co-ordinators to be supported in maintaining contact with the many strands of service provision that may need to be drawn together to form an individual's integrated care pathway.

While some care co-ordinators will be offering treatment or specific care/support as part of an integrated package, others will need to adjust to a care co-ordinating role that is at times more akin to case management. This may not come easy for some healthcare professionals who are used to being the treatment provider. This also highlights the importance of clarity as to who offers care co-ordination and how will health, social and criminal justice services be organised into a genuinely collaborative process. Is care co-ordination primarily a healthcare function, and, if not, at what point does it become more of a social care responsibility?

Treatment modalities will need to be clearly defined, and individuals' roles and responsibilities in terms of service provision will also need careful definition to ensure everyone works within their own sphere of professional competency. Also, what is being offered needs clearly defining so that a client referred in for a particular form of treatment or support can be sure of what they are being offered and its appropriateness to their needs.

Most of all, perhaps, we should focus on the service users, the people for whom the service exists. The challenge of Models of Care lies in ensuring that the client is placed at the heart of service provision, that it becomes a genuinely client-centred system. The danger is that they will be squeezed into 'one-size-fits-all' care pathways based on diagnosis and predetermined, rigid protocols. But for the system to work holistically, to ensure that the needs of the person are met, then each care pathway will be tailored according to client need and expectation, individual care plans reflecting the uniqueness of each person's needs. As it is stated in Models of Care, 'Good systems of care planning and care co-ordination will ensure that services are client-centred' (NTA, 2002, p. 39). This, if it is achieved, will ensure a revolution in drug service provision.

PART 2

The patient's journey through Models of Care

CHAPTER 2

'I don't have a drug problem'

- Hospital ward (Tier 1) Level 1 assessment
- Hepatitis B, C and HIV interventions (Tier 1)
- Drug outreach (Tier 2) Level 2 assessment
- Referral to Tier 3 service for Level 3 assessment

Monday 15 May – intensive care ward, local hospital
Mark could hear sounds around him, voices, footsteps. He could smell warmth, and other smells that he couldn't really distinguish, it was the warmth that he was more aware of. But he was not aware of feeling warm in his body. In fact, he didn't feel aware of his body at all. Just sounds and smells.

He had no idea how long he had been laying there; in fact, he had no concept of laying. No spatial sense at all. He tried to concentrate on the sounds, trying to distinguish the voices, but he couldn't, and they began to fade, it seemed as though they were becoming distant. There was a kind of buzzing sensation all around where Mark was experiencing the impressions that were affecting his auditory and olfactory systems. It got louder and then silence. Nothingness.

The nurses continued their routines, unaware that Mark had begun to gain some sense of the world around him. Nothing had stimulated the battery of monitors to which he was connected. They were as oblivious of his presence as he now was of them. He had lapsed back into unconsciousness.

It was well into the next day when Mark again began to experience a sense of the world around him. Voices again, blurred and distant, and the smell, he knew that he was familiar with it but couldn't place it. He felt strangely heavy. He was aware of his body now, not of any sensations other than the sense of heaviness, of not feeling able to move. He could sense his eyes now but he couldn't move them. He tried to force some movement but he couldn't sense anything happening in his hands.

What had happened? Where was he? Mark struggled to think clearly but he could feel himself fading once again. His body was heavier, he felt heavy in his consciousness, and once more he slid back into unconsciousness.

Tuesday 16 May
It was later the next day when Mark was able to open his eyes and he could feel his body. He began to flex his fingers, he was able to turn his head and he looked

across to the doorway. He felt awful. What had happened? He could remember getting some gear [heroin, though sometimes used to refer to injecting equipment]. Yeah, he could remember going to the dealer and getting the smack [heroin]. Some new stuff, the dealer'd said. And then going back to his mates' place, yeah, he could remember that.

He wasn't on his own, that's right, Nick and Paula had been with him. And now? Well, he was clearly in hospital. He swallowed, his throat was dry, and irritated by a tube that was down the back of his throat. He coughed; it attracted someone's attention. It wasn't long before other people had arrived. They were asking him questions, and telling him to take it easy. They told him he had overdosed and that he was lucky to be alive. That he had been lucky. His two friends had noticed the signs and called for an ambulance straight away. They had fortunately been on an overdose prevention training course which a local drug service had been offering to users. They'd seen him go over and had had the presence of mind to put him into the recovery position and get help. But he had still gone unconscious and had been out for a few days.

> Overdose rates associated with drug use – illicit and prescribed – is a key area for development within services.

During the next few days, as Mark began to gain his strength and his focus, the staff began to talk to him about his life and his drug use, seeking to take an interest in him, in what had happened, and to encourage him to recognise the dangers associated with his drug use. Mark was shocked by it all; it was the kind of thing he never really believed could happen to him.

He was still on a detoxification regime, now gradually reducing what he was receiving.

Mark had listened to all the arguments about the dangers of his drug use and, yes, he heard what was being said, but deep down he knew he was going to use again. It was such a part of his life, himself, it wasn't something he was contemplating changing, whatever the risk. So he'd overdosed, yes, but he'd survived. He was good. He wanted to get out and get back on with his life.

> The fact that someone has experienced a life-threatening event does not mean that person will automatically feel motivated to change their drug use. Some will, many won't.

The staff were clear that having identified a drug problem in a patient, as a Tier 1 service, they referred them on to a Tier 2 service so that someone could engage with the patient and undertake a more detailed (Level 2) assessment. The local statutory service which offered mainly Tier 3 services but also co-ordinated drug outreach services (Tier 2) within the area decided an informal contact would be the best first step. Mark had been recognised as an injecting drug user and so one of their drug outreach team was nominated to make first contact with Mark, try to get to know him, start to assess his level of use and any damage done and begin to offer harm reduction advice.

As part of their own protocol in response to having an injecting drug user on the ward, they had carried out tests for hepatitis B and C, with Mark's agreement. He'd turned down an HIV test – didn't want to know. He was clear of both types of hepatitis, but they then offered to vaccinate him against hepatitis B. He agreed to it. Nearest thing he'd get to a needle for a while. And, yeah, made some sense the way they'd described it.

Basic harm reduction intervention: checking to see what hepatic disease there is and then minimising the risk of catching an hepatic virus (B) in the future – there is no vaccination for hepatitis C although it is widespread among injecting drug users. Mark is lucky, very lucky, not to have it.

Phil arrived, dressed in his usual gear – couple of rings in his left ear, tattoos up his arms, black T-shirt, faded jeans. Turned a few heads as he walked down the wards. Phil was used to that. He knew the scene. He knew he shocked a few people but he wasn't here for them, his job was to engage with Mark, and the way you dressed, the way you talked, the way you walked, all said something. Mark was struck by the contrast between Phil and the staff on the ward. Well, he could hardly miss it! He wasn't in the least bit 'medical' as some of the other staff, and seemed more chatty. Seemed to know his way around the drug world, and spoke Mark's language. Phil asked how long Mark had been in and what had happened. Mark said what he could remember. Phil nodded, bit of eye contact but not too much. Keep it informal, keep it loose.

Not every outreach worker, or indeed drug worker, is like Phil. He has his own particular style. Outreach workers come from a variety of back-grounds, but in general they need to be good communicators and be able to reach drug users (not that there is necessarily a stereotypical drug user either). They seek to reach out, as their role suggests, make contact, communicate, get information and advice over to the drug user, seek to encourage harm minimisation and harm reduction attitudes and actions. They may work with more chaotic clients who have not got to the point of feeling ready to refer themselves into a more structured drug assessment and treatment programme. So they may attend a drop-in, or it could be the outreach worker goes out to people – in their homes, perhaps, or to meet them on the streets. They may be providing injecting drug users with clean needles and syringes and offer advice on safer injecting techniques. What they offer may also be governed by their own professional background. Some outreach workers are generic drug workers; others have nursing backgrounds, or counselling.

It might be unusual for an outreach worker to go on to the hospital ward in this way, but it can happen. Perhaps a nursing intervention might have been more helpful, maybe not. Sometimes ward medical and nursing staff will handle the medical response to a drug user on the ward.

'So, I suppose you'll go out and jack up again, yeah?' It was said in such a matter of fact, non-condemnatory way that Mark was taken aback.

Up till now he'd been telling everyone that he wouldn't use, all the staff – doctors and nurses who had asked him about his drug-using intentions – as much to stop them going on at him as anything else, get them off his back. They had all seemed to want to tell him that the only answer was to say 'no' to drugs. But with Phil, he somehow felt a little less guarded. But he still said 'No.'

'No? Most people do. Threat of death doesn't always stop people.'

'Well, not me.'

'OK. Great. So you're going to make some changes then in your life, yeah? Keep some distance between yourself and your suppliers and the guys you've been using with.'

'I'll be OK.'

'Yeah, I'm sure you will, but I want to level with you, Mark. People don't stop using just because of the kind of experience you've had. Some do, but some don't – many don't. I may not be able to stop you using, but I can talk to you about what options you have, to try and keep yourself safe, you know?'

'I'll be OK.' Mark sort of liked Phil but he was irritating him. Seemed to know a little bit too much.

Phil noted Mark's defensiveness and backed off. He knew there was little point in pushing him where he didn't want to go. He well recognised that pushing a person often made them dig their heels in, and made it harder to maintain some degree of authenticity in the relationship.

'I hope so, I really hope it works out for you.' Phil was aware – the staff had told him – that Mark's veins were pretty messed up. They reckoned he must be having trouble getting a vein up. Phil decided to use this to try to get alongside Mark. He was concerned. It was clear to him that Mark was saying he was OK but clearly wasn't thinking it through and didn't have much of an idea how he would try and remain drug-free. In fact, he wasn't at all sure that Mark was motivated in this. He seemed too off-hand about it all.

Mark didn't reply. He wanted Phil to go away. He was feeling better now, just wanted to get out of the place and get some relief. Yeah, he needed to jack up, knew he'd feel so much better.

'You've been injecting a few years I gather so I guess you're pretty skilled at getting a vein up, yeah? There are techniques for this, to make it safer, you know, and ways to inject to reduce the risk of damage. And of course, clean works [injecting equipment], cuts back on the infection risk.'

Mark heard what Phil was saying but he wasn't really interested. He'd get by.

'Don't want to hear any more. Why don't you fuck off and bother someone else?'

'That what you want?'

'Yeah. Want a bit of space.'

'OK, I'll give you a bit of space.' Phil sought to empathise with Mark and just leave it open, hoping to have communicated that he is hearing what Mark is saying that he wants, hoping that through this he can begin to build a relationship between them that will lead to Mark trusting him and being more ready to listen to him.

Mark snorted to himself. He said nothing.

Phil respected Mark's silence.

'Here are details of where you can call me, and here's some leaflets about injecting smack, the risks and what you need to know to minimise doing yourself more harm than good. You may find them useful. We can offer you advice, information, clean works, but I can tell you about all that another time. It's in this leaflet though.' Phil knew that the ward planned to keep Mark in for a while, so he knew he'd have time to follow up his informal contact. He could see Mark wasn't someone who seemed particularly ready to give up.

Phil put the leaflets down on the bed and got up to leave. 'I'll drop back later in the week, see how you're getting on.' He looked Mark in the eye. 'You look after yourself.'

Mark held his gaze for a moment before looking away. 'Yeah.'

Phil has sought to engage with Mark, but Mark doesn't want to know. He decides rather than to keep pushing him, he's left contact details and some information. He has sought to be respectful to Mark, to not get into a heated discussion over the pros and cons of his drug use. Other staff have clearly spelled out the risks. Phil prefers a different approach. Spending a little time with the client, trying not to be too pushy, seeking to remain professional, clear as to what he wants to communicate to Mark, but ready to adjust to where his client is in himself. Phil has sought to show respect to Mark, but has also given him information and an opportunity to think about what he is doing and consider a safer approach. He hasn't undertaken a formal assessment at this stage; that can follow. Mark is in a safe and supportive environment.

Friday 19 May

Mark was feeling better physically as the week went on but he was feeling churned up inside. Lots of memories in his head from his past; he was finding it hard to cope with the feelings that he was experiencing. He'd always used substances since his early teens, stopped him feeling good, bad, stopped him feeling.

He didn't like what he was experiencing, he wanted to get away from it and the only way he knew how was to get some gear. He couldn't talk about it. He felt sure that would just make it worse, and, besides, talking wouldn't take it away, just make you more aware of it. He wanted his drugs, shit, how he wanted to experience that beautiful relief and release. Even the thought of it made him feel a little calmer. Yeah, he'd get out as soon as he could, say the things they wanted him to say, and then get back into his life.

Phil came back in as he had promised later in the week.

'Hiya, still here then?'

'Yeah.'

'How're you doing, mate?'

Mark nodded. 'Yeah, feeling good.' He wasn't, but didn't want to get into that.

They were sitting in the common area. Mark certainly looked better, had a better colour and just looked healthier. 'You're looking good. Eating well?'

'Yeah. Not used to eating much but yeah, a little.'

'So, what are your plans. Any news as to how long you'll be in?'

'Rounds tomorrow. Making a decision then. They're referring me to your drug service, want to me to talk to someone to co-ordinate my care. I don't need to be cared for. Fuck's sake.'

'Mhmm, want to get on and live your own life, yeah, don't need someone caring for you?'

'No, fucking don't. Bloody care something or other. I don't need caring for, that's for kids. Told them I'm OK, not interested, but they're making the referral anyway, and, well, we'll see.'

'Mhmm. Care co-ordinators aren't there to kind of mummy you, you know. More to make sure you get any services that you need.'

'Doesn't seem like that to me.'

'Well, I'd suggest you give it a go. I mean, I'm part of the package too, it's a matter of working out with you what you want, what'll be helpful, and making sure it's made available to you in a way that you can access it. At the moment, well, we need to discuss what you want. In fact, it's unlikely you'll be allocated a care co-ordinator straight away, depends what your needs are. I mean, you might decide you just want some advice, clean works and informal contact with me. But you might want more than that, perhaps seek to go on a methadone programme, and maybe other interventions and support as well. So, I know they said care co-ordinator, but really at the moment we're looking at building up an initial assessment to ascertain your history, current drug use, needs and how they can best be met, and what treatment services you might need/want to be referred to. We can then move on to a more comprehensive assessment at the drug treatment unit, with a doctor and nurse – specialists in drug issues.'

Care co-ordination within Models of Care will only be offered in case of complexity where structured Tier 3 treatment responses are required. To begin with, Mark needs an initial or Level 2 triage assessment. Out of this will

come a recognition of whether the client needs, and is seeking, a comprehensive Level 3 assessment. Should the comprehensive assessment take
place, then a care co-ordinator will be nominated who will then co-ordinate
a pathway of care in which the different treatment modalities are integrated
and centred around meeting the client's needs. Once Mark's needs are
agreed, and knowing what treatment modalities are available, the integrated care pathway can be formulated for Mark.

'So what might they offer, then?'

'Well, as I say, maybe you might want substitute prescribing, for instance, if
you go back to using, or feel tempted to but don't want to inject or use off the
street. Or maybe you might want counselling, or relapse prevention support.
Or group work. Maybe some social work input. There are lots of options. The
assessment back at the unit will help you to decide what is going to be helpful,
and enables us to get a clearer, more in-depth picture of the situation.'

Mark was listening but got suddenly bored, and switched off. 'Yeah, well, not
interested. Rather find my own way, stick with my mates, you know.'

Phil was still feeling sure that Mark was planning to use, and he really wanted
to make a connection with him, begin to build some kind of working relationship,
and get some more clarity as to what Mark needed. He didn't want to get
embroiled in a formal assessment, but he knew that it was important to assess
his needs and at that moment he, Phil, was the only drug specialist engaging
with Mark. It seemed appropriate for him to at least get more background information and then encourage Mark to have a more formal, Level 3 assessment,
depending on what seemed appropriate. He hadn't completed the Level 2 assessment, he'd taken what he had learned from his conversation with Mark and filled
out the assessment form but there were gaps. However, he realised that Mark was
unlikely to engage at this time in such an assessment. Nevertheless, he asked
some questions about how long Mark had been using, what substances, family
background, whether he'd had any mental or physical health problems and
what treatment he'd had. It was clear that his drug use had been for a few years
and that he hadn't had any mental health problems diagnosed. What he had
gleaned, however, had made it clear that Mark was likely to need some form of
substitute prescribing if he ever decided to address his opiate use. The prescribing
clinic was at his service and would be part of the integrated care pathway formulated for Mark if that was what he wanted.

These are the levels of assessment referred to in the introduction. Mark has
been given a Level 1 assessment within the hospital (which also offers a
Tier 1 level of intervention). Phil, however, can begin a Level 2 assessment
and begin to get a sense of Mark's level of need and any complexities and risk
factors that will need addressing further by healthcare specialists, or by
other professionals, for instance, social workers. His outreach work is a

Tier 2 intervention although the statutory service he works for offers treatment modalities within both Tiers 2 and 3. In this instance the decision has been taken for an outreach worker to begin the process of engagement. Other services might well have sent in a substance misuse nurse to undertake a more formal assessment – either brief (Level 2) or comprehensive (Level 3). Some hospitals/drug treatment services have dedicated liaison workers/nurses providing the necessary liaison links between services. In this instance, the client is being referred into the substance misuse clinic for further assessment.

'So, I know you've had an initial assessment which included stuff around your drug use, the fact that you have been injecting, messed up some of your veins, which was enough for them to contact us, yeah, but it'll be really helpful for me to have a little more background. And maybe then we can help you, whatever you want to do about your drugs. I mean, I know the gear is important to you, yeah, and there's a good chance you'll go back to it. And I know you're saying you won't, and great if you don't, but I know the score. I've been in this game too long to believe everyone is going to stop using when they say they'll stop, yeah? But if we can help you avoid using, or choose to use in a way that's less harmful, well, I'm up for trying to make that happen, you know?'

'Yeah, well, I can hardly tell you I'm going to start using, I mean, you'll have them stop me getting out.'

Phil shook his head. 'No, that's not how it works. I know that if you really don't want to stop then I can't make you stop, none of us can, you know that. Let's get real. Yeah? You've used gear a long while now, and it's part of your life, a big part. OK, you're detoxing here, well, you've detoxed now, haven't you? You're clear, clean, and yes, that's an opportunity, a chance for change. I'd like you to take that chance, make that change, and we can support you and encourage you in this. But if that's not what you want, OK, that's your choice. I think it's a less healthy choice, yes, but if that's where you're at, so be it. I'm not encouraging you to use, but if you're going to let's be sure you're doing it safely and you don't wind up back in here or worse, yeah?'

Phil is trying to ensure authenticity. He knows that unless he can level with Mark it is unlikely they will be able to really connect over Mark's drug use, and an opportunity will be lost. Phil knows it may take time, it may not happen now, but if he can at least earn Mark's respect then there may be a doorway left open for him at a future time. However, at the moment there is an opportunity. Phil wants to use it and encourage Mark to take it.

'Yeah, I don't want to be back here again.'

'Well, look, the word on the street was that the stuff you used was a bit purer than what you're used to, and stronger, yeah, some new batch and you reacted.

It was too much. And when you go out now, you aren't going to be able to use like you have been. You need to keep the level low for a bit, adjust to it. Yes?'

'Guess so.'

'You don't want this happening again?'

'Guess not.' Mark was shaking his head.

'OK. So, first of all you need to decide what you're going to do. Want to carry on seeing me, taking time to talk about things a bit? Work out just exactly how much you can use and avoid the risk of overdose again?'

'Yeah, but I'm not gonna stop. I mean, maybe one day, but not yet.'

Phil notes Mark has now said he's not going to stop – he notes it to himself but doesn't make a big issue of it. Just lets him know he's heard him. He keeps the contact and the conversation flowing. Too many searching questions could put Mark back on the defensive and an opportunity will be lost.

'OK. You're going to use. You've had a health check, blood tests?'

'What for?'

'Hepatitis B and C.'

'Yeah, I'm OK and they're vaccinating me against hepatitis B.'

'And you're clear of C?'

'Yeah.'

'You're lucky, need you to stay that way. If you're going to inject again, you've got to have clean needles and syringes, yes, and we can sort you out for that. It's important.'

Information about hepatitis risk should be a standard procedure among drug services, whatever tier. Hepatitis B vaccination programmes are a Tier 1 service. Information about HIV and hepatitis C should also be available across tiers with referral on for treatment to specialist services.

'OK.'

'Look, you're young, give yourself a chance, Mark, what are you now?'

'I'm 23.' Mark paused. 'I can't see a life without the gear, you know, I mean, can't see it.'

'Mhmm. Hard to imagine when you've never experienced it.'

'Yeah. It's like, oh I don't know, I get confused. Using the gear makes me feel OK, you know?'

'Yes.'

'You say yes, you ever used?'

'Yes, I did, long time ago. Got clean, gave myself a chance of a different life, and, well, here I am I guess on the other side of the fence. But, yes, I know it's difficult, hard to believe you can change, but you can, people do, but it's hard to do it on your own. The rewards, though, are better health, less serious risk to yourself – and you're here because of one of those risks – having a life not spending all your time organising the next fix. How many years do you want to carry on like that? Two, five, ten, longer? Is that what you want?' Phil was deliberately seeking to help emphasise the negative effects of continued use, seeking to help Mark engage with some degree of motivation or desire for a different life for himself.

Mark shook his head. 'When you say it like that, no, I guess maybe not.'

They continued the conversation, Phil gradually gleaning more information about Mark's drug-using past, his recent pattern of use, how he got into it. Eventually he made the point of reflecting back what Mark had told him, and how, yeah, he could offer him help and support, and that he could be referred for an assessment for a more structured programme if that was what he wanted. But if he didn't that was OK; he could still access a range of services and support, but more informal.

Tier 2 interventions, as described in the introduction, will be more informal although with a primary drug focus. Mark is a client at a crossroads and more than anything what is important is that he is encouraged to maintain contact with services. If that means the informality and unstructured nature of a Tier 2 intervention then that is what needs to be offered. Appropriate care pathways must be made available for Mark. He needs information as to who to contact and where, and Phil can offer a useful advocacy role if needed, as well as general and specific outreach support.

In mentioning the less structured and more informal approach, while this has many plus points for engaging clients, it can also lead to boundary problems. Many, though not all, drug users struggle with boundary issues. Edges are blurred. It can leave both the professional and non-professional stepping out of role. The need for quality supervision is vitally important when working with this client group. To put it another way, drug use can leave people living in a very different frame of mind, and in the attempt to understand that experience, the person working with them can themselves feel blurred, adopting some characteristics of clients, in effect generating a kind of parallel-process experience. This can also happen in teams; for instance, the 'quick-fix' mindset of clients – particularly early in recovery – can induce similar attitudes to problem solving within the service.

'I haven't mentioned it before, but ever consider going in to a residential rehabilitation unit, you know, going in somewhere to kind of get your head straight around everything?'

'Nah.' The thought made Mark feel anxious. Bloody hell, locked up, no drugs, all touchy feely, shit, he'd heard about that stuff. No fucking way, he thought to himself. He'd heard how tough some of them were too, being torn apart in groups. Not bloody likely, he thought. No way.

'Just a thought, now that you're clean, you know, could seek funding, get you in somewhere if they can hold you here while the funding is sorted out.'

Mark was shaking his head. He was feeling very anxious all of a sudden. He felt like he was being trapped into something. No way. No fucking way, he thought to himself.

'OK, but I wanted to at least mention it as an option. So, you're being referred for a comprehensive assessment with the team, they can then work out with you what will be the best package of treatment.'

Level 3 assessment is appropriate for complex cases, high risk/need, mental health problems, and likelihood of the client not engaging with services. This will include medical as well as psychiatric assessment and history.

'Treatment? Makes it sound like I've got some disease. I don't need treatment, I need some good gear, set me up, make me feel good again, yeah?'

Phil could sense that Mark was suddenly getting more agitated. 'You're on edge, yeah?'

'All this talk about treatment and rehabs and stuff, shit, so I used a bit too much, yeah, I'll be more careful next time. For fuck's sake, give me a break, man.'

'OK. So, where do we go from here? You going to attend for the assessment if you're offered one?'

'Maybe.' Which as far as Mark was concerned meant 'no'.

'Or do you want a less formal support, like a drop-in and, well, meeting up with me, and maybe a support group to help you if you want to try and stay off.'

'Nah. I'll maybe use clean works, you know, yeah, that makes sense. Now I know I'm clear of those infections. But it's OK, I mean, it's OK to have 'em?'

'Sure, come up to the clinic. We also give out containers to put the used works in – reduce the risk of sitting on a used needle, you know – or someone else picking it up and using it ...'

'Uhuu.'

'And, look, injecting, you see the booklet I left?'

'Yeah. I've been doing it all wrong, haven't I?'

Phil encouraged Mark to describe his injecting technique. Yeah, he was right, it wasn't too good. He showed him how to do it to minimise the risk of damage. He didn't inject anything, just showed him the angles, and explained the danger of injecting in certain parts of the body, and in particular to keep away from anywhere near arteries. Phil gave a good graphic description of a needle in an artery.

'You on the level?'

'Yeah, can happen, and believe it's a mess, and you don't need it, do you?'

'Shit, no.'

'OK. Look, let me know when you are discharged. You still got my number on the leaflet?'

'Yeah. And I did look at them cartoon leaflets as well. Bloody funny. Yeah, saw myself in some of them characters, you know? Had to laugh.' Yeah, he'd had to laugh. Kept the other feelings away, it had.

Phil encouraged Mark to tell him of his history of drug use, and his family background. Thought he might be able to fill in a few more of the gaps in the details the hospital had passed on and the Level 2 assessment he was putting together. Mark was reluctant at first, but Phil made it sound like it was safe to brag a bit about what he'd done. And that led him into a little about his background.

'OK, so, I've got a clear idea of your use in the past, yes, and some of the crap that's happened in your life. I'll keep in touch with you. Got a mobile number I can call you on?' Phil decided to increase the likelihood of maintaining contact with Mark.

'Yeah, can't use it in here though.'

'No, but when you're out and about we can keep in touch, you know, informal, yeah?'

'Yeah, OK.' Mark was still feeling anxious about all this treatment stuff. He didn't want treatment. Just wanted to get on with his life. Maybe he'd be better off not staying in any longer. He was up and about now. They'd talked about discharging him soon, but wanted to know where he'd go to. He said he could stay with his mum. The hospital seemed OK about that. Phil had only been with the service just over a year; he didn't recognise her name as an ex service user.

Karen had been assigned the task of offering Mark a comprehensive assessment for his drug use, and she had contacted him on the ward to say she would come over to have a chat with him early the following week. It was preying on Mark's mind. He didn't want rehab, he didn't want 'treatment', he didn't want to be 'cared for'. He wanted to get back to the gear, but be a little more careful in future. What did they say, lightning never strikes twice? Yeah, he'd be OK, just be a bit more careful. Ease up on his use. Not use quite as much, take it steady for a bit.

His discomfort and unease grew over the weekend and it was Sunday afternoon when he could stand it no more. He discharged himself. Went round to his mate's and scored later that evening [scoring – using drugs, generally refers to injecting]. Yeah, he was more careful and, yeah, he used clean works. Turned out that his mate Pete had started getting works from the needle exchange since Mark's overdose. Paula and Nick, who had found Mark when they'd got home, had also been given information about overdose. They'd been friends of Mark for a while now, given him support when he was dealing with a lot of hassle during teenage years. They actually knew him from when he was a kid, and were happy to give him a place to sleep. They knew the history and the difficulties he had. They had both used drugs a little in the past, but hadn't been there for a long while now. They did enjoy a few drinks though and, from time to time, smoked a little cannabis, usually as part of a social get-together.

They'd been in to see Mark, and had also tried to get him to think about what he was doing, but he wasn't thinking about that. They'd also got information on overdose – the paramedics had given them the contact number of the local drug service.

Summary

Mark has overdosed. The people he was with had fortunately received training in overdose prevention and recognised the signs. This training was offered by a local drug service that offers both Tier 2 and Tier 3 services to clients. The overdose leads to Mark being admitted to a local hospital, Tier 4b, where he is given specialist care. An outreach worker, Phil, makes contact with him and seeks to persuade him into treatment, but Mark isn't interested. Phil seeks to engage with Mark, offering him harm reduction information and seeks to establish an informal connection. He applies motivational techniques to help Mark realise that he wants his life to be different, and to help him realise that there are other options. Phil raises the idea of a more comprehensive assessment but Mark is uncomfortable about this. The weekend before Mark is due to have his comprehensive drug and alcohol assessment he discharges himself from hospital.

CHAPTER 3

Engaging with the drug service

- Needle exchange (Tier 2)
- Referral to Tier 3 service for Level 3 assessment
- Prescribing clinic (Tier 3)
- Assigned care co-ordinator (Tier 3)

Monday 22 May
Phil had learned that Mark had discharged himself when he came in to work on the Monday. He had tried calling Mark but had not been able to get through. Seemed that probably he hadn't paid any money into what was probably a pay as you go phone. Mark had given his mum as his next of kin, and had said that he could call her if he needed to. While Phil hadn't appreciated the history, Karen had as soon as she saw the assessment form. She had been at the service a bit longer and could remember Mark's mother being maintained on a methadone script [colloquialism for 'prescription'] herself for a number of years. She'd been reducing down when she'd first joined the team five years back, and had held it together quite well as far as she knew.

Phil felt that he needed to try and make contact with Mark. Yes, he respected his right to choose to discharge himself from hospital. Yet he also wanted to try and ensure that there was minimum risk. He knew it was a risky time – people going out and using after they have detoxed which would have happened to Mark while he was in.

But he hadn't got permission to call Mark's mum. A dilemma. He couldn't breach confidentiality. Did Mark's mum know about his drug use, or that he had been in hospital? In one sense he knew he was experiencing an urge to reach out, find out what was happening, or at least give himself a chance of this. And yet confidentiality was confidentiality. He didn't have Mark's permission. He discussed it with Karen and they agreed to send a letter to him, coming from Phil as he had had the initial contact, asking him to make contact.

Monday 5 June
A couple of weeks later Mark comes in to the needle exchange one afternoon. Phil happens to be around. He offers him a coffee and they go and have a chat. Mark's been living partly rough, partly at a mate's house that's more of a squat than anything else. He hadn't got the letter straight away.

He'd nearly been caught shoplifting: 'Needed to score, had to grab that fucking radio, didn't I, didn't know it was chained down. Fell over the bleeding TV in the shop and they nearly jumped me. Bastards. Just got away.' He paused. 'It's been bad, haven't had much money, scoring now and then but not enough, you know? Need to do something about it. Also need some clean works as well. Started to use 'em, can see the sense in that. Pete's using them now, and, yeah, the people I was living with, they'd encouraged me too.'

'OK, so any idea what you think you want from us?'

'Guess I want a script, you know, guess I need to go on the meth, something to hold me.'

'OK, so you're looking for a methadone prescription, is that right, oral?'

'Guess so.'

'Supervised consumption, you know that?'

'Yeah, I know, stop me selling it on, I know.'

'Also makes sure you take it, you know, so you're getting a consistent dose. One of the reasons for prescribing it is to take out some of the chaotic haphazard use. Lowers the risk of overdose so long as you don't use on top.'

'Yeah, OK, so, what do I do?'

'Well, we have a prescribing clinic [Tier 3 intervention] but we need you to have an assessment here with the doctor who prescribes and one of our team. We can get that organised for you by the end of the week. We'll need a urine sample, one now would start the ball rolling, and we'll need another before we can prescribe.'

The urine sample will enable the clinic to check whether the substances that a client claims to use are in fact being used. Once the person is receiving sub-stitute medication, ongoing tests can check to ensure that the client is not 'using on top', in other words, using other substances on top of that which is being prescribed. Where this is happening it could be that the client is not receiving a high enough methadone dose to keep them stable. Alternatively, they might be selling it on (if there is no supervised consumption). An aim of substitute prescribing is to bring greater stability into a person's drug use, as well as reduce the harm they might be otherwise doing to themselves. Giving a urine sample should, where possible, be supervised. It is not unknown for a client to have a container with someone else's urine to fill the bottle they have been given. The first obvious check, when given a urine sample for processing, is to see whether the bottle is warm!

'OK, I can probably pee now. Didn't have one before I came over.'

'OK, so let's get that sorted and then we'll get an appointment organised, yeah?'

'OK.'

Mark peed into the bottle, with Phil watching on through a small hinged flap in the wall. It took him a while. Never seemed to pee too freely these days. He put the top on the container and handed it to Phil who had held out the bag to put it in. Phil then took down some more details – what had been happening since Mark had discharged himself from the hospital, building up more of the picture. He checked Mark's address – he gave Nick and Paula's – 'best place to get in touch'. He asked if there were children living at the house. Mark shook his head, 'no'.

Phil again checked on Mark's level of use – hadn't gone back up to what it had been before he'd been in hospital. He'd let the doctor decide on the prescribing regime. Wasn't going to get into talking amounts. Phil checked the appointment book – there was a slot for Friday morning.

'Friday, 11.00am. How's that?'

'Yeah. Thanks. You were right, I can't go on like this, got to give myself a chance of changing. Been a rough couple of weeks.' Phil encouraged Mark to talk about it. 'You know I discharged myself?'

'Yeah, wondered what that was about?'

'Thought of treatment and got it in my head I'd be put in a rehab. Just got out of control, had to score, you know. So I got out. Yeah, I needed it but, well, I've been drifting around, scoring when I can, nicking stuff, drinking, dossing around, couple of nights on the street when I was really out of it. Can't cope with it, you know, need to change.'

'Out of it with the gear, or . . .?'

'Hit the alcohol when I couldn't score. Nicked a few cans, and spent time with the guys on the street, who meet up in the park. They shared some of what they had. Good on 'em. But they're where I'm heading. Mum had a go at me when I turned up there last week. Rowed with her. Did my head in, you know?' He breathed a heavy sigh. 'So, need something, can't go on like this. Fucking skint again, but Nick and Paula are back now so I'm going to see them. Haven't seen them since I came out – they'd buggered off to some festival somewhere.' He paused. 'So, Friday, yeah, can't do anything before then?'

Phil shook his head. 'We need the urine tests. And we need you assessed by the doc. But he'll sort you out on Friday. And you'll be allocated a care co-ordinator who'll probably be at the consultation as well. Can't say who just at the moment. That'll be organised at our referral meeting on Wednesday.'

'OK, thanks for that. Can I have some works before I go?'

Phil sorted him out with what he needed. 'Tried phoning you, couldn't get through.'

'Yeah, money ran out on it. Have to get more added.'

'You going to be able to get over here on Friday?'

'Yeah, no problem. You be around?'

'Can be. Will that help?'

'Yeah.'

'OK, I'll see you then.'

Friday 9 June

Mark arrived for his assessment. He'd got the time wrong and had arrived half an hour earlier and had to be persuaded to wait. He complained that he had to be somewhere else and he couldn't wait. The receptionist had noted his problem but had remained assertive about the appointment time. It was then that Phil arrived. Mark tried to persuade him that he needed to be seen right away. Phil reiterated that the appointment was for 11.00am. He didn't want to undermine the receptionist by trying to let Mark be seen sooner. He'd seen how some clients could pressurise people and the clinic here was very clear about time boundaries. The drop-in was informal, but booked appointments had set times and that was that. Besides, he knew that the doc had other appointments; the door was closed so someone else was being seen. He encouraged Mark to wait. Mark wasn't too accepting of this. He continued to remonstrate with Phil who was very conscious of how different Mark was in contrast to when he had last seen him.

'What's got to you, Mark?'

'I'm fucking clucking [withdrawing], man, haven't scored since yesterday, fucking clucking. Feel fucking awful man, and if I can't get anything I'll have to go and get a can, something, anything, man.' Mark was pacing up and down. 'I need something now, man, fuck it, can't you do anything?'

Phil took the decision to take Mark out of the waiting room. Whatever the truth of the situation, he felt he could contain things better in a separate room. As he ushered Mark towards one of the consulting rooms he spoke to the receptionist. 'Tell Dr Ashton as soon as he's free that Mark's here, says he's clucking, desperate to see him. I'm in room 4 with him. OK?'

'Yes. Glad you came in. Can't get on with anything when someone's like that.'

'I know. I'll try and get him settled. Thanks.'

Mark gradually calmed down although he was clearly on edge. Dr Ashton finished early with the previous client and buzzed the phone to let Phil know he was free. Phil went through with Mark into the doctor's room. Helen was also there; she was a specialist nurse and would co-ordinate Mark's care.

'So, Phil mentioned you'd been in earlier in the week and we've had a copy of the discharge summary from the hospital after your overdose, yes?'

Mark nodded. 'I'm feeling bad, doc, I really need something.'

Dr Ashton explored with Mark what his symptoms were.

'I need a script, doc.'

'Looking for a methadone prescription, is that right?'

'Yeah.'

Dr Ashton continued with his assessment procedure, referring to what Phil had already written into his more brief assessment, checking in more detail on the client's level of use, his history of use, physical health – symptoms, injecting sites. He took a mental health history – there wasn't much for Mark to say. He hadn't overdosed before, no suicidal ideation. Family history? Yes. His mum had overdosed a few times in the past.

The medical assessment and treatment might be carried out by a GP with a specialism in substance misuse running a GP-led clinic, or it could be a psychiatric doctor. Services vary in terms of the nature of the specialisms for medical input.

He reaffirmed that it was on-site consumption, and that it would be dispensed over the weekend through a local pharmacy where consumption again would be supervised. Told him he needed to know exactly what Mark's level of use had been, double checked it again, and warned of the danger of him talking up his usage. Agreed that he would be started on a 30 ml dose, that he should take that now, but stay around for a while for it to take effect and see how he was feeling later in the afternoon. He didn't want to over-prescribe, but he wanted to be sure he was prescribing enough to hold him. He also said that, in view of his level of use, he'd probably eventually refer him on to the GP Liaison service offering Tier 2 interventions and would discuss the prescribing with his GP, but that would be once his use was stable. For now the consumption would be supervised at the clinic on a daily basis, and later could be moved out to the pharmacy who also supervised consumption. They would make that decision later if necessary. Dr Ashton also indicated that he would write to Mark's GP so that he was aware that Mark was receiving methadone from them.

Good practice. Minimises the risk of 'double-scripting', where a client gets one prescription from one place and another elsewhere.

Dr Ashton warned him about using on top (where a client uses more of the same substance or other substances on top of what is being prescribed – potentially dangerous and lethal), that there would be random urine tests to check on what was in his system. If he used then they would want to discuss it, that they couldn't prescribe if he 'messed about with the gear'. 'We will have to review your script if you use, Mark, we aren't in the business of encouraging the risk of overdose.' If he felt he was at risk of using on top, Dr Ashton encouraged him to make contact with the service, and indicated that Helen would give him a range of helpline numbers for support out of hours and at weekends.

Mark nodded. He seemed pretty easy going, and, yeah, he seemed to give it to him straight. Well, he'd have to see how he got on. Mark thanked Dr Ashton and Helen organised the on-site supervised consumption.

'That wasn't so bad?' Phil commented as they left the assessment session.

'No. So, I see Dr Ashton weekly?'

'Yes. And I have to shoot off, but I'll leave you with Helen.'

'Thanks.' He turned to Helen. 'So, what now?'

'Well, I'd like to see you early next week to check out how you're going with the methadone, and to talk through what options there are for you by way of other forms of support and help. I'll be seeing you weekly, for a while at least, and we'll monitor how things are going. And you'll see Dr Ashton, and I'll sit in on those sessions as well. The next appointment with him will be next Wednesday. But what I need to do with you next week is to sit down and work out a care plan with you. We touched on some of it just now, but it would be good to spend more time looking at options, yeah?'

> A documented care plan makes clear what the client, and the service, are agreeing to. It will be reviewed regularly – and this can be done formally or informally – to ensure that what is being offered to the client remains pertinent and appropriate to their needs.

'Yeah, OK.'

They arranged a time. Helen had another appointment to attend to. 'We'd like you to wait around in the clinic, be sure that the methadone is holding you but not over-sedating you. Another member of the team is on duty and I'll put him in the picture. His name's Barry. He'll come out and have a chat. I can make you a coffee or tea if you like before I go.'

'Yeah, coffee'd be great.'

'And there are some magazines and stuff around. But I'll let Barry know you're here and he'll come and have a chat.'

Helen went off and returned with the coffee. Barry had already sat down with Mark and they were chatting. She gave Mark his coffee and collected her bag before heading off. 'See you Monday, Mark.'

'Yeah, thanks. See you then.'

Barry stayed with Mark for about 15 minutes and then a call came in that he needed to attend to. He took it and came back out 10 minutes later. He checked how Mark was feeling. He said 'good'. Barry let him know that he was still around if he needed him.

Mark was feeling easier as the methadone kicked in. It left him feeling a little sleepy but not too much. It was midday and he wanted to head off. He asked the receptionist if she could let Barry know. He came out, checked him over, checked how sleepy he felt, but Mark said he was OK. He'd see how he was getting on and would call in later if there were problems. Barry asked if there was anywhere where he could be reached, but there wasn't. His phone was still out of money. Barry made it clear that if he experienced any problems, if it was within working hours, to call the clinic, otherwise the GP.

> Not ideal, but the pragmatic reality is that not all clients of drug services will be contactable. The question is whether this means they are not entitled to treatment. The supervised consumption ensures containment in terms of the level of use of the prescribed medication. The client can still go and use on top, but they could do that wherever they were. At this stage it is important to ensure the client is getting what they need to hold them.
>
> Where the dose is high, there is a need to titrate the actual dose taken to ascertain what is required. While this is best done in an inpatient facility to monitor levels of withdrawal or over-sedation overnight, this is not always available.

Monday 12 June
It was time for Mark to arrive for his appointment and Helen was looking at the clock. It wasn't unusual for people to be late. She sat back and waited, flicking through the assessment that she and Dr Ashton had completed the previous week. She could see that his problem was going to be time. He wasn't using, so he didn't need to spend time stealing to feed his habit, or time to score.

Time. So often the problem. No doubt Mark would need some structure in his life, some kind of routine. But it was her experience that so few of her drug-using clients could manage time and structure. They were often normalised into more chaotic lifestyles. They tried to be informal but keep to structures in the service. Bit of a blend of Tiers 2 and 3 in many ways. Sometimes that could be difficult within a service; clients could be confused. Outreach and drop-in were informal, and some of the support groups had a certain informality about them, keeping clients in contact with the service. Then there were the more structured groups, the day programme and the one-to-one therapeutic counselling. And, of course, appointments with her and the doctor. She tried to be as flexible as she could, but there were limits. She rarely did home visits except where there was a real issue about access to the service – severe disability, or mental health problems limiting a person's ability to get out.

Ten minutes had passed, no sign of Mark. Strange, he hadn't been in for his daily methadone; she had assumed he would take that after her session with him. That was usually a good enough motivating factor to get people to attend, at least to begin with. She hadn't a number for him, only his friends Nick and Paula's address. She decided to wait out the session and if he had not arrived to send a letter first class reminding him of the appointment, offering another appointment – she could see him later in the week – and confirming that he had to attend as part of the prescribing agreement.

Mark did not arrive and there was no message from him. She sent the letter.

Services need protocols as to the timing and content of letters to clients who do not attend an appointment. However, form letters may not encourage people as effectively as more personalised letters. While the latter may take more time, this is efficient if it encourages clients to re-attend or at least make contact. The wording of letters can be hugely significant, often having the potential for significant therapeutic impact on clients.

Wednesday 14 June
Mark did attend the appointment with Dr Ashton who was aware that Mark had not attended his appointment with Helen. She had, however, organised to see him immediately after his appointment with the doctor.

Mark explained what had happened. He'd got into an argument on the Sunday with his mum. Said he needed some money to buy some food – he actually needed it to get some gear – and she'd refused to give him anything. He'd been taking his methadone and all had been OK. But, he didn't know why, he'd just felt weird that afternoon. He'd felt himself craving. Tried to fight it, decided he needed to score. Went to his mum for money, there'd been a row, he'd got really angry and had taken money from her purse, pushing her away when she'd tried to stop him. He was really shocked; he'd never done that before and didn't understand why it had happened.

> The urge to use can be overwhelming to the degree that nothing stops the user from getting what they need for their next fix.

He'd then carried on using on the Monday. Knew he ought to come in for his methadone but thought he'd blown it, and so bought some on the street. But he knew he couldn't go on like that; it was just going to take him back into his chaos. So he'd come along today, say what had happened and hope he could continue with being prescribed.

'We need you to try not to use on top, Mark. We know it's difficult and we know it happens. And we do need you to attend these appointments and we realise that there are times when it's not easy. We have to keep in touch with you, Mark; each time we see you it's like an ongoing process of re-assessment, checking out. We're trying to help you stabilise and we can't do that when you're not using consistently. Was it that you needed more methadone?'

'I was OK Friday and Saturday, it was Sunday that got to me, and I hadn't planned to use Monday, but, well, I had the money by then and, well, you know. Coming off Sunday night's use, well, I just did it.'

'Yeah, OK, but you need to talk through with Helen what happened on Sunday to see if there is something that can be planned to resolve it. And what about your mum? Things can't be good there either.'

'No. Haven't been round since. I feel bad about it, I really do. That's not me, not to my mum.'

'Surprised by how angry you were?'

'Yeah, I mean, I really was angry, and I don't know what that was about. She pisses me off sometimes, always on edge, she unsettles me, always has.'

Dr Ashton thought about anger management but he also knew that often managing anger didn't necessarily help the person get to the root cause of the anger. 'So something caused the anger and it got taken out on your mum.'

Mark nodded. 'Guess she knew why I wanted the money. There was food in her flat, I could have had that if I wanted food. She's been there, she knows. That's why she said no.'

'And you exploded.'

'Went crazy. Still feel angry but more with myself, you know? But why did I go crazy? I was really suffering, you know, why couldn't she have let me have some money. Bitch. If she'd given me enough just to score once I'd have been OK, but I took more, and, yeah, well, had to use it again and again.'

'Mhmm. Injected?'

'Yeah.'

Dr Ashton went silent and looked across at Helen. Helen asked Mark how angry he was now. She was wondering whether the methadone might be stopping the feelings breaking through that perhaps his pattern of heroin use in the past had kept at bay.

'Still angry. Well, I mean, not angry but, uptight, you know, does my head in, yeah?'

'Yeah. I guess we have three options here, maybe four. First, carry on with the current script and get you to monitor your mood, particularly your anger. The second option is to increase the dosage on your prescription, though that's the one I least favour. Just a quick fix and we want to break the cycle of quick fixing, Mark. Third option, same script but look at anger management. Fourth option, maintain the script and refer you to therapeutic counselling to try and resolve the cause of your anger. And you may have some other ideas, Mark?'

Upping the script sounded attractive. Just take it all away. But the doc had already made it clear he wasn't too happy with that. Counselling was an option, someone to talk to. He did feel that maybe that might be good. Someone to talk to. He didn't have many people he could really talk to. Well, he had Nick and Paula but they ... well, he didn't want to load them up with his stuff. They'd been good to him. But he also didn't know what counselling would feel like. Anger management, was that what he wanted? He knew he had to control what he was feeling. He'd never been good with feelings. 'Can I think about it? You're not going to give me more methadone, are you?'

Dr Ashton was shaking his head. 'You're not withdrawing, are you?'

'No, I was OK on it until Sunday. Then I used the gear. Stopped on Tuesday, ran out of money. And I knew I had to come here today, needed to get my head straight.'

'OK, so you want to think about it. Talk it through with Helen.'

Dr Ashton gave him another prescription for daily supervised consumption and Mark left the session and went into the room opposite with Helen.

Given the treatment being offered, and the range of needs that Mark has, Helen now begins the process of exploring what else will be most helpful to Mark. She also confirms herself as his care co-ordinator.

'We need to look at what is going to help you, Mark. My role here is going to be that of co-ordinating what we offer to you. First of all, though, we need to be clear as to what exactly you feel you need so that we can see what treatment interventions we can match to your needs. Where do you want to begin, Mark?'

'I dunno. I'd love more methadone.'

'Yeah, I'll bet!' Helen smiled as she said it, holding eye contact with Mark.

'But that isn't going to happen, is it? Your doc's pretty clear on that.'

'Yes, he is. We can't start giving out methadone to control emotions that are not associated with withdrawal reactions. We need to know what you're angry about.'

Mark took a deep breath. 'OK. Well, my father pissed off when I was ten, my mother took up with this other guy who hated me, got excluded from school 'cos I kept being disruptive – hit one of the teachers, took to drinking on the streets then using the gear, and here I am, fucked up. Lots to be angry about.'

'And you feel that anger now, I mean is it anger in your heart, your head, in your guts?'

'It's in my head, I guess, though it's everywhere too. But I don't think about these things, I think about, you know, what happened Sunday, how my life is, you know. Haven't really been angry, I mean, not really angry – too much time out of it I guess.'

'What about when you were in hospital and detoxing, were you angry then? Was that why you left?'

'I was angry that I might have to go into rehab, that I was being seen as some-one needing "treatment". I just want help, I'm not ill, I just want help.' At this Mark's eyes welled up with tears. He closed them and swallowed. 'Oh shit, sorry. I don't do that.'

'You don't cry?'

'No.'

'Seems to me like you have a lot of strong feelings you are bottling up and maybe, just maybe, they've been controlled by your substance use over the years, but now that you're trying to control that some of these feelings are get-ting out. Anger broke through when you detoxed. Maybe you've a lot to feel angry about?'

Mark nodded. 'Makes sense I suppose.'

'So, what option do you want to take?' Helen did not want to tell Mark; she wanted him to decide on what he felt was most appropriate for him.

'Guess it's the counselling, isn't it?'

'I think so. I'm not a therapeutic counsellor. I can use counselling skills in my work as a nurse, in offering support to you and helping your motivation to change, but I think you need something that goes deeper, that can help you to, well, get in touch with yourself in a safe environment, in touch with the stuff that maybe the gear's been keeping at bay. Yes, you need to learn to manage the anger, but maybe that will be resolved by you getting it out of the system to some degree.'

Mark nodded. Yeah, he knew he had lots of stuff in his head, that sometimes he just couldn't cope with it and used the heroin to just get away, get some relief.

Helen was continuing. 'And besides, I have to keep an overview to co-ordinate what we're offering you, and you need to maybe talk things through with some-one who hasn't got responsibility for your script. Seeing someone for your feelings and thoughts, clear of the medical stuff, is more likely to be helpful.'

So, as care co-ordinator, Helen is now organising for Mark to not only receive medical and prescribing responses from the doctor, but now therapeutic counselling as well. Two care pathways but they are integrated – medical/prescribing and therapeutic – with Helen's role being to ensure that what is needed is available and accessible to Mark.

'So I see someone to talk about these things, and how do you fit in?'

'Well, as well as having a medical role, I'm your care co-ordinator so I ensure that what you need is being offered. I re-assess your progress, if you like, provide a focus within the service, and we may decide that other interventions or support would be helpful and I would be the person to help ensure that the "care pathways" that you are offered are appropriate to your need.'

'So, I still see you?'

'Yes, we can work out how often.'

'And how often would I see the counsellor then, and who is it?'

'We have counsellors in the team and I don't know how soon. There may be a short wait; I can check that up and let you know. Have you got a phone I can contact you on?'

'Leave a message with Nick and Paula. I'm going to stay at their place for a while now. Call me there or leave a message. They know I'm coming here.' He gave Helen the number.

Helen presented Mark with other options that he might want to consider: the day programme although that was geared more for people who were stopping their use, a drug awareness and education group, an informal support group for people who were struggling at different stages with their drug use, contact with a social worker to maybe look at his social needs.

'Think I'll take it slowly and start with the counselling. Not too sure about groups.'

They discussed this and decided to leave that option open. She wondered about getting him to see Phil, but in way he'd done his job, bringing Mark into the service. They wanted to try to establish some structure to Mark's week, with appointment times. Ideally, a community support worker would be good, but they didn't have one. Helen raised her concern about how Mark was going to use his time, particularly if Nick and Paula were out a lot of the time.

'They don't, not much. A bit. But not when I'm around. They're really supportive. They use cannabis more than anything, but not much.'

'And you mentioned last week that you use it as well.'

'A bit, not much, trying to use less.'

'So, your time?'

'Watch TV, videos, need to get a job, I guess.'

'Mhmm. We've got links through the local college to an initiative that gives people work experience and helps them develop skills. It's run in conjunction with the local technical college. I can give you a leaflet and, if you want, set up a meeting with one of the staff.'

'I'll take the leaflet and think about that. I do need to use my time, I need to move on, do something with my life, get out of the craziness.'

'Yeah. OK. I'll get that for before you leave.'

Helen mentioned the idea of a kind of mood or anger diary that Dr Ashton had sort of mentioned. 'Might help us get a handle on what's going on. You could use this diary, it has columns for mood.' She handed Mark an A4 sheet with columns and rows on it. Time of use, period of use, mood before, amount used, mood after, cost, comments. 'One row per day.'

'OK, I'll give it a go.'

The rest of the session was spent looking at Mark's next week, helping him to plan his days. Helen agreed to let him know how long the wait was for counselling and Mark left after having taken his methadone.

Mark's current care plan is for him to continue with daily supervised metha-done consumption and weekly contact with the prescribing doctor.

Thursday 15 June

Helen phoned Mark the next day; she caught him in and was able to tell him that he could begin the counselling in three weeks if he wished, and that he would be seeing Tony.

Mark thanked her and said that he did feel he needed to go for it, that he needed to take the opportunities that were available, and that he also wanted to look into the work training she'd mentioned. Helen agreed to take that forward and they could discuss that the next week.

Summary

Mark misses his appointment having used at the end of the weekend and over the period when his appointment was booked. Issues related to anger have emerged and he is offered structured therapeutic counselling (Tier 3 intervention), which he accepts. He also agrees to vocational training (Tier 1 intervention). He continues being prescribed methadone (Tier 3 intervention).

CHAPTER 4

Alcohol and referral on for more support

- Methadone maintenance (Tier 3)
- Care co-ordination (Tier 3)
- Structured therapeutic counselling (Tier 3)
- Referral to day programme (Tier 2)

Monday 19 June
The follow up with Dr Ashton the following week was on the Monday and was uneventful. He had switched him to his Monday clinic where he had a gap in his booked appointments. He'd fitted Mark in on the previous occasions in space he kept for emergencies. But he wanted to offer Mark a stable appointment time to start the process of helping him towards structure in his life. Mark had managed to stay with his methadone during the week, hadn't used on top, hadn't much to say really. Dr Ashton insisted on a urine test, explained it was procedure, that they would test at random, reminding Mark that it was part of the agreement they had. Mark reluctantly agreed. At first he said he couldn't pee, so the doctor pointed him towards the water dispenser. Mark drank, but kept insisting he couldn't pee. Dr Ashton held to his demand and, eventually, Mark did provide a sample which was sent off that day for testing. Mark took his methadone before leaving. He wasn't due to see Helen until the Wednesday. She was on a training event and was not available until then.

Wednesday 21 June
Mark came in to see Helen. She asked how he was, whether there had been any particular problems and enquired about whether he had been able to track his mood since she had last seen him.

He said that he had calmed down again, made things up a bit with his mum, though it wasn't easy with her at the moment. He realised that he'd been feeling guilty about his drug use for a while, and Helen asked him how he dealt with it.

'Guess that's one of the reasons I use. Crazy. I use, feel guilty about it, and then use again, and so it goes on.'

Helen could see a clear cognitive-behavioural cycle running. 'So you perceive your drug use as something to feel guilty about, and that's uncomfortable so it triggers drug-using behaviour and then round you go again?'

'Yeah. Been like it for a while.'

'Mhmm, always driven by feeling guilty about using?'

'Not sure that I really mean guilty.' Mark thought about it for a moment. 'More ashamed really. Guilty about what happened the other week, yeah, but generally it's about feeling ashamed, you know? I mean, I remember as a child thinking, shit, I'll never be like mum, you know, having to use. I mean, from early teens I was aware of what was happening. Christ, the flat was a tip looking back, didn't want to be like her, and I am.' He went quiet.

Helen decided to pursue it a little further. She didn't want to get into anything deeply therapeutic, the counsellor would provide that opportunity, but it was a theme with Mark at this moment and it seemed appropriate to maybe help him make sense of it.

In her care co-ordination role with Mark, Helen is using counselling skills. There are times when it may seem, in reading the dialogue, that she enters into more of a counselling mode. Sometimes it is not easy to keep the two apart. Care co-ordination is a relational process and it is going to contribute to a therapeutic effect on the client who is being helped to understand their drug use, their choices, their difficulties, and be encouraged to maintain their motivation. One of the big challenges that Models of Care throws up is that of defining the role of the care co-ordinator, and how this role might be embraced by people coming from different professional backgrounds. In some settings a care co-ordinator will be actively offering 'care' or 'treatment'. Elsewhere this may not be the case; their role will be strictly one of co-ordinating 'care' and 'treatment' offered by others.

'So it was pretty chaotic and you intended not to be like mum, yeah?'

'And here I am, a junkie. At first I tried to keep it from her, but, well, word gets around, you know? She was angry with me at first, threatened to throw me out, but she couldn't really, I was only 14 at the time, you know?'

'Tough time, yeah?'

'Yeah.' Mark lapsed into silence. They'd been bad times. His mum's boyfriend hadn't been much help. He used as well, but it hadn't been through them that Mark had started. It had been through some guy outside the school on the estate, he'd been giving it away. Group of his mates had a go, Mark didn't think he'd get hooked, knew he wasn't like his mum, wanted to see what it was all about. And, yeah, it had been good, fucking good. He'd just felt so clear of everything in his head. Hadn't realised how different he could feel. Started smoking and kept with it for a few years. He'd convinced himself because he smoked smack it wasn't like his mum, who injected. But it didn't last. He'd got into injecting when he'd got that job down by the docks. Met up with a different crowd and, well, he gave it a go and, yeah, felt so good, reminded him of those early days when he'd started chasing, only better. But, well, you know the rest.

Helen asked if he wanted to talk more about that period in his life, but Mark shook his head. Said no, upset him too much, made him feel things he didn't like. She asked if he was still OK for the counselling, and he said he was, he wanted to give it a go, but he wasn't sure it would help. Helen suggested that he give it a few sessions at least and see how it worked out.

They turned to the mood diary that Mark had been keeping. Most days he'd felt low, some days more anxious than others. He hadn't really felt angry that much, more on edge really. Helen asked him how he coped with the difficult days, with the anxiety. Aware that he'd used on top when he'd got angry, she wasn't sure how he'd handle anxiety.

'Try to keep away from it, you know? Have a few cans, that's what I tend to do. I mean, I have in the past but usually didn't need to, you know, I'd be using the smack to do that. But, well, the meth doesn't really hold me, well, it sort of does, you know, but I do get anxious at times and, yeah, couple of cans helps.'

'Couple?' Helen wanted to just double check the amount before moving on. 'Couple' was such an easy thing to say, but didn't always mean 'two'!

'Mostly, not always, sometimes I didn't, but on a couple of occasions I had more, about four.' Mark was beginning to feel a bit anxious himself now, talking about this.

Helen noted the anxiety and decided she needed to clarify further the 'about' but also acknowledge the fact that he looked a bit uneasy.

'You don't look too comfortable talking about this, Mark, and while I want to acknowledge that, I do need to check the "about" as it is important for me to get a sense of exactly how much you are needing to quell the anxiety.'

'Well, yeah, six one day. Didn't feel good about it, helped but left me feeling ill next day.'

'What, physically ill?'

'Yeah, threw up and just felt so groggy. Only recently really been using the alcohol like this, I mean, like I say, before I could get the gear, you know, that kept me together. Now, well, it's difficult.'

'Mhmm. I guess what we need is a discussion with Dr Ashton on this. I mean, we'd rather you tried to keep to one substance, you know. It's difficult, alcohol's legal and, you know, you've got a right to drink if you want, but if you're drinking to cope with stuff that maybe the methadone could help with because it's linked to your reaction to coming off the gear . . .'

'Yeah. More'd be great.' He grinned. 'But it's not that simple, is it?'

'No. We need to explore whether your experiences really are linked to the withdrawal, or whether you are reacting to specific triggers that could be managed in other ways. But I have to be clear that it is dangerous for you to drink alcohol on top of methadone. It increases the suppressant effect and can, in particular, lead to a suppression of the respiratory system, and can lead to people being at greater risk of vomiting and choking. It really isn't good news.'

Mark nodded. He was aware that in fact it wasn't just alcohol he'd used. Damned urine test yesterday, he wasn't sure what it might pick up. He sort of thought it was just for opiates, check he wasn't using heroin on top. But he wasn't sure. He knew he'd used benzos a couple of times, got them from a friend on the street. Wasn't much, he kind of thought that they wouldn't show up. He'd pretty much convinced himself it wouldn't show up.

Benzodiazepines are tranquillisers and, as with alcohol, exacerbate the suppressant effect of the methadone, putting people at risk. The urine tests ensure that the prescribing doctor has a clearer idea of the chemical cocktail they are dealing with. Unfortunately, many people develop a parallel dependency with benzodiazepines.

The session continued with Helen seeking to encourage Mark's motivation. It was a hot day and it felt heavy going. Mark seemed distracted, and she mentioned this. He just felt low. She explored this with him, wondering if there were signs of depression, but it seemed more likely it was fatigue. He hadn't been sleeping too well, hadn't really slept well since stopping the heroin.

It was clear from the mood diary that Mark was feeling quite flat at times, and yet he was also experiencing the anxiety. Part of the problem was the chemical adjustment, and also the effect of the methadone, but also Mark simply wasn't used to having a body that was not strongly affected by suppressant chemicals. The methadone wasn't being prescribed to 'take him out of it', but simply to hold him, help him get clear, get a different structure and routine to his day, and then it could be re-evaluated. At the moment, though, Mark was struggling to feel motivated towards anything at all. Spent a lot of time in bed, watching TV, just finding it hard to adjust. He didn't like the flatness in his mood. Well, he did in a way, but he was getting bored with it.

Mark agreed to carry on monitoring his mood. He didn't bring up the vocational training – he hadn't actually given it much thought. When Helen mentioned it he said that maybe he would later, but not yet. Felt he had too much going on, too much to sort out in himself.

He agreed to try to get out a little but he highlighted how he found it easy to stay in – didn't like bright sunlight too much. Helen suggested if that was a problem, how about sunglasses, would that help? He hadn't thought about that. She sought to encourage him to give it a go, try and at least help him acclimatise a little to being out, to get some fresh air rather than be indoors all day, other than getting out for his methadone and a little bit of shopping. Said he wasn't eating too good, and they also looked at strategies to help with this, identifying which foods Mark might feel more able to eat, and which at the moment should be avoided because they'd put him off.

Mark left feeling a little more motivated to eat, and, yeah, he'd liked the idea of trying the sunglasses. He knew he wanted to change, but shit, it seemed hard going.

Monday 26 June

The test result had come back, and it was positive for benzos. Dr Ashton confronted Mark. 'The urine test's back, Mark. I guess you know what it's showing.'

Shit, thought Mark. Do I act innocent, claim it must be a mistake? He knew that wouldn't work, and anyway, he didn't want to mess things up for himself – well, he realised he already had.

'Yeah, well, I got anxious and couldn't settle and my mate had some diazepam, and, well, yeah, I did, but only twice.'

'OK, but we do need to be real with each other, Mark. We're trying to help you adjust to life without heroin, and we want to try and get you stable on the methadone. I'm not going to prescribe benzodiazepines, let's get that clear.'

Mark felt a sudden burst of anger. 'No-one wants to fucking help me. You don't give a shit. I need my drugs, I feel fucking crap, you know? You don't, you don't know what it fucking feels like. Shit.' Mark got up and moved towards the door, then hesitated – what was the use in walking out? But he felt so angry.

'You're angry, Mark, and, yeah, it's bloody tough going. We want to help, and we need to work at it together. I know that sounds a bit of a cliché but we do. We've got to help get you stable, and we've got to help you get on top of the anger.'

'Haven't been angry much, not till now. I mean, shit, I need help, man, it's fucking hard out there.'

'So we need to work with you to find out what can be done to get you through this period, yeah, without it all getting back out of control.'

'I don't want to use other stuff, I don't, but it's hard, shit it's hard.' Mark felt the anger being replaced by despair. He knew he wanted to change, had to change, to get a better, different life. He'd spent so long around drugs, they were in his head, they'd been that way for so long; if he wasn't taking them, they were around him at home. He was so fucking tired of it all. But he couldn't get them out of his head.

Helen responded first. 'We'll look at the options after this session, Mark. I'm wondering whether we ought to see about you attending that day programme the non-statutory service runs; maybe it's more important for you to have structured support each day, get a routine together. Maybe we were expecting too much to suggest you could hold it together with the methadone, weekly meetings with me and Dr Ashton, and one-to-one counselling which should start day after tomorrow.'

Mark didn't know what he wanted, just knew it felt like a nightmare. He shrugged.

It was Dr Ashton who responded. 'We've got to get you stable, Mark, if that's what you want.'

Mark nodded. 'Yeah, I can't go on like this, I can't.'

'OK, but we need to formulate a plan that will really help you. What's the hardest part of it all at the moment?'

'Sitting around, trying not to think about using.'

'OK, so time's a big factor, yeah?'

Mark nodded.

'So maybe, Helen, we need to see about the day programme, and if that doesn't work, maybe you need more contact here, Mark, and then we'll review it.'

Assessment has to be ongoing, and will require modifying of the care plan. Mark's need for time, focus and structure had again been highlighted as significant. It is also clear that this structure may need to extend beyond the agency that Helen and Dr Ashton work for. The day programme is offered by another service and therefore there is a need for co-ordinated and integrated inter-agency working. Helen, as care co-ordinator, will be responsible for organising this and ensuring lines of communication are open. It will involve integrating another care pathway into Mark's package of care, and may require adjustments to ensure access.

'Guess so.'

'I'll find out about the day programme, Mark. In fact, maybe I'll try and do that now while you finish this session with Dr Ashton.'

They agreed to this and Helen went off to make the phone call.

'Hi, Helen from CDAT [Community Drug and Alcohol Team], wondering if I can talk to someone about a client of ours? Yeah. He's new to the service, on a methadone script, struggling to hold things together, needs more contact, more structure with his day and we're wondering what you could offer through the day programme.'

From the conversation it was clear that there had been some recent changes to the programme, that they could be flexible, that in fact they were planning another group which would be for people still using and seeking to be in more of a maintenance phase than abstinence. They'd found that there were too many people wanting maintenance and the abstinence-only group wasn't offering enough. As a result this second group was being commissioned.

Helen asked what the programme offered and basically it wasn't going to be every day to start with, but twice a week, Mondays and Thursdays.

She got the information she needed and went out to find Mark.

'Hi, come on through. I've spoken to Carrie who is going to be involved in running the programme. It's not starting for about a month. They're planning to start it the beginning of next month – Mondays and Thursdays, for people who are using and trying to maintain control. It's a new programme, and seems ongoing. They'd like you to see one of the group facilitators before the start, to get to know you. They can take the assessment we've already done, so no need to go through all that again, but they think it's good for participants to meet one of the facilitators before the first day.'

'What do they do?'

'Some of it's group stuff – helping you look at behaviours and how you think about things. It'll help you get a better understanding of how you think about things and how that leads you to make particular choices – like use, or what triggers anxiety, anger and so on. Be an opportunity to learn from others as well, and it'll give you a bit of structure to the week.'

'What about seeing the doc? I see him on Mondays.'

'I'll talk to him about that. He has another clinic here on Fridays and we can switch you across, I'm sure. We'll have to think about your methadone script as well. Their programme starts at 10 o'clock and so you'll need to take it here before you go on to them, or maybe switch to taking it later afternoon, after the programme. They're aware you'll be on a script. They're gearing up to work with people who are going to be substance-affected, but hopefully stable enough to engage with what they're doing. I think they're also planning to build some other skills training as well – getting you to cook meals together, things like that.'

'I guess the thought of having it before the programme would make it easier for me, but I'd probably be better off having it after. I guess I need to change my routine.'

'Yeah, you want to try and take it consistently each day around the same time if you can.'

Mark was aware of feeling anxious again at the thought of it all. 'OK, I'll give it a go. No promises, mind, not too good in groups, but I've got to do something.'

'Guess that's why you haven't used NA [Narcotics Anonymous]?'

'They need you to stop, you know, I'm not there. They want you to be clean and, well, I'm still using the meth.'

'Well, this programme is designed for people who, like you, are trying to maintain themselves on methadone. I guess, though, we need to look at the next four weeks. You start the counselling Wednesday, maybe if you see me on Thursday as well during this period and we'll see how it goes?'

'OK, I can tell you about the counselling. Want me to keep with the mood diary?'

'Was it helpful?'

'Yeah, helped me be more aware of things. But, well, I'm still not sure if I can hold things together, though I know now I can't use the benzos. But I do want to keep control of the alcohol.'

They looked at the drinking pattern and other options Mark might have to relax and unwind. It was clear that it was the evenings that were difficult. Seemed that the others where he was living would tend to drink some evenings and Mark would join in sometimes. Helen again pointed out the dangers associated with drinking alcohol while taking methadone.

'I can't ask them to stop.'

'No?'

'Well, I mean, if they want to drink, I mean, they're free to, you know?'

'Mhmm, and maybe if they appreciated what you are trying to achieve, maybe they might change their habits, perhaps?'

'Dunno, doesn't seem right, somehow. I think I'd be better off going out.'

They explored where Mark might go. It turned out that Nick and Paula had a dog, and so Mark decided he'd suggest taking it for a walk. It didn't get many walks and maybe that would be good for him to do. The dog's name was Henry. So, little did Henry know but he was about to experience a more healthy lifestyle.

Before Mark left, he apologised for getting angry earlier. 'Just felt like everyone was getting at me. I'm trying, Helen, I really am, but it's fucking hard going.'

Helen nodded. 'Yeah. We'll help you get there, Mark, you can do it, just feels like you can't sometimes.'

Mark left. He was feeling more positive. He'd got some ideas. Next thing, the counselling, Wednesday afternoon. He wasn't sure what to expect exactly, but he knew it was likely he'd be expected to look at his past. It wasn't a place he liked to go. But he knew as well that he needed to talk to people and at the moment it felt that the more people he could talk to, perhaps the better he might feel. At least he could get things off his chest.

Summary

Mark continues to attend his appointments with Dr Ashton. He is taking his methadone but has used benzodiazepines – which came up on a urine test – and alcohol to quell anxiety and feeling on edge. He is working with a mood diary to help him better understand himself and what triggers mood change. It is recognised that he may need more than one-to-one counselling. He is referred to a non-statutory agency which is soon to be starting a day programme for people on methadone maintenance or any drug that they are seeking to maintain control of their use. Mark's alcohol use also becomes clearer, but rather than increasing the methadone it is decided that more support and contact and other diversionary strategies might be more helpful. However, the position is to be kept under constant review.

CHAPTER 5

Counselling begins, preparing for the day programme

- Methadone maintenance (Tier 3)
- Care co-ordination (Tier 3)
- Structured therapeutic counselling (Tier 3)
- Day programme waiting list (Tier 2)

Monday 3 July – prescribing clinic
The next appointment with Dr Ashton was routine. His follow-up urine test to the one that had shown the benzodiazepines had been clear. Mark said he felt glad he was seeing Helen the extra day. Gave him something to hang on to during the week. He said how that was really how it felt at the moment, as though he was just hanging on, holding himself together as best he could. He mentioned that it was a little difficult coming to the clinic for his methadone – tended to bump into people he knew were using on top, and some were dealing. They agreed that he'd spend time talking this through with Helen to review the options; however, they did discuss changing the medication. Dr Ashton introduced the idea of Mark switching to Subutex (buprenorphine). It reduced the risk of overdose. Mark had heard about it, and what he'd heard was while it was easier to take, it didn't give you that cloudy feeling. He wasn't sure about making the switch. Dr Ashton made it clear that he needed him to try to ensure he didn't drink too much, and possibly not at all, while on the methadone.

Subutex contains buprenorphine and while it is classed as an opioid medicine it is suggested by the manufacturers that it does not have such a strong effect on the brain as heroin and methadone. It is a tablet available in three different strengths, and it has to be dissolved under the tongue to have an effect. It can be used to stabilise as well as for controlled detoxification.

Care co-ordination
'Yeah, it isn't easy, you know, coming here each day. Just run into too many people and it's like it's good to see people, yeah, but it isn't good as well.'

'Really uncomfortable, good and not so good.'

'Yeah, and it's like, you know, if they're hanging out when I leave, I don't really want to get into too much conversation and yet I also want to, you know? I feel quite isolated at times. I mean, yeah, they're using the gear and stuff but they're my mates too.'

'They're important to you, but . . .'

'Yeah, but . . .' Mark paused and thought back to an incident the previous week. 'I mean, last Friday, came in to get the meth, you know, and there was Stuey, yeah, we used to spend a lot of time together, and, yeah, he's . . . don't suppose I should say this, well, anyway, he's still into stuff, you know, and he started talking about it, wanting to meet up and stuff. And yeah, we had good times together, but, I dunno, it was tempting, you know, made me think back.' Mark went silent, nodding his head as he thought back to the past.

Helen felt it would be helpful for Mark to clarify this past experience. She knew how often it might be thought about as positive but actually the reality could be different. People often hold on to beliefs about their drug-using past, kind of reminiscing about how it was, particularly when they are in the process of trying to make significant changes.

'OK, so it brings up thoughts for you of how it was, good memories, huh?'

Mark nodded. Yeah, he thought, they were good. Well, most of them were dominated by using, so it was a bit hazy, except for the drug use. Yeah, like it all ran into itself.

'Any particular memories?'

Helen is seeking to help Mark clarify exactly what his memories are. If they are not as good as he makes out, then she can help him to perhaps accept a different perspective which may help motivate his change and help him cope with these difficult incidents. If the memories turn out to be genuinely good ones then they are definitely relapse triggers and then need addressing from that perspective.

Nothing particular stood out. 'Just using, you know, getting off together.'

'So the memories are more about the drugs than about Stuey?'

Mark thought about it. 'Dunno. Hadn't thought of it like that.'

'I guess I'm wondering how much Stuey played in your memories and how much it is the effects of using.'

'He was around.' Mark was thinking back. It hadn't always been easy with Stuey. Bit of an arsehole at times, he thought to himself, did crazy things, he'd been the one first got him into jacking up, showed him how to inject. Yeah, that had been a good time. Mark was back in the experience. It had never been as good again, not after that first one.

Helen noticed that Mark seemed to have drifted away into his own thoughts and it seemed to her that he was smiling as he sat there.

'You look miles away, something nice to think about?'

'Hmm? Oh, yeah, sorry, yeah, thinking about Stuey. Well, and about using. He started me injecting. Yeah … and you know, in a way I still feel glad for that, and another part of me wishes I'd never met him.'

'Mhmm, and which one is the greater?'

Mark thought about it, and it was the memories of the smack that dominated his thinking. The problems, even the overdose, weren't to the fore. 'For real?'

'Yeah, for real.'

'The smack, the feelings that it gave me, such wonderful, wonderful feelings, just floating away from it all, from everything, from the stuff in my head, from memories, from hassle, from everything.' He took a deep breath and let it out slowly. 'Still haven't cracked it, have I, still got too many good memories about it.'

'Yeah, but it's good to recognise it, you know, we know what we're working with. We can focus more on relapse prevention and that's going to come up in the day programme too, and I guess we can begin preparing you for that by starting to look at that now and over the next few weeks.'

Mark was looking distant again. 'There's just nothing quite like it.'

'Mhmm. Unrepeatable experience?'

Mark nodded. 'Yeah, never did recapture the first feelings but then, well, it was still good, and then, well, had to have it, you know, felt so bad without it.'

Helen was still concerned in her own mind with helping Mark separate out his feelings for Stuey and those for the heroin.

'And Stuey introduced you to it, yeah, at least, got you injecting?'

'Yeah. Took me to another level, you know? Real good. Didn't think I'd stay injecting, thought I could control it, yeah, but no, I couldn't, had to use again, and again, just took me away from everything so beautifully, kind of silky somehow.'

'Mhmm, so, as you've said, smoking heroin since aged 14, then into injecting a few years back. And Stuey got you into injecting. And now it's difficult seeing him because he's still a mate but you don't want to get caught up in his world again.'

'No, I don't. I mean, yeah, it was good, really good. But it got bad, real bad, yeah? Out of control. Nicking stuff to feed the habit. Shit, full-time job keeping myself together, you know? Crazy days. Glad it's over though.'

'So you're glad that what Stuey introduced you to is over, yeah?'

Yeah.' Mark could feel anger, and it was towards Stuey. Bastard, he thought. 'Can't keep seeing him, you know?'

'Does it make you want to use?'

Mark thought about it. 'Not exactly. I mean, no, I don't think about using and yet he starts talking about the old days, and, well, it sounds so good, you know, so much easier than it feels now.'

'All that nicking and hunting down a dealer, and jacking up, yeah, and having to do it, having to 'cos you feel like shit if you don't, much easier than it is now?' Helen knew she was deliberately being provocative, wanting to help Mark get clarity around what he was saying.

'Not when you say it like that. But, I mean, I didn't feel like I had any worries. I knew I could get stuff and, yeah, it wasn't often that I was clucking for too long, you know?'

'So you'd go back to those times, then, given a choice, they're that attractive?'

'No.' Mark paused. 'No. I can't. It would kill me. Got to move on.'

'OK, so you're clear, you've got to move on. The heroin felt good, you loved it, and you love to think about what it felt like, but it's no good any more, yeah, and you don't want Stuey kind of encouraging you to think positively about your drug use.'

'No. He's still full of it, full of shite, bastard. He'd get me back using tomorrow if he could, you know? Doesn't give a fuck.'

'He doesn't give a fuck,' Helen paused, 'but you do.'

Mark nodded. He was thinking. Yeah. He did give a fuck. That overdose, at the time, yeah, he was still intent on using, but now, now that he was thinking about it more clearly, fuck, he could have died. It could happen to him. It had happened once, and it could happen again. In fact, if he'd used on his own that time he might not have made it.

The harm minimisation response is that injecting drug users should not use on their own; they are at greater risk of overdose. Hence the importance of raising awareness of the signs and symptoms of overdose, and how to respond, within the drug-using community. Often they will be the first people to notice someone is having a problem, and they can therefore reduce preventable deaths.

Helen sat with the silence. Mark looked as though he was thinking. He didn't seem to have drifted off this time.

Mark looked up. 'I have to change so much, Helen. You know, I almost wonder if I need a fresh start, somewhere else.'

'Is that realistic?'

'Got a cousin in the south west, he's often said if I wanted to get away I could go down there. He's got a big place on the coast. Maybe that's what I need.'

'Mhmm, can see yourself getting away from the area and from your contacts.'

'May be the best thing. But I'm not going to rush into it. Though maybe I could go down to see him, but then again, what about the daily methadone?'

'We can work around that, maybe if you plan a specific length of time we can organise with a pharmacy down there for you to pick it up. We can talk to the local drug service to see what the situation is. Now that we have teams around the country working to the same standards, and with the similar services, it shouldn't be a problem. But we need to plan it, think it through.'

With drug services working to similar standards and levels of service provision, arranging for someone to be out of the area and yet continue to receive their methadone in a controlled way – daily, supervised consumption – becomes possible. It would be possible for him to take a number of bottles, one for each day's dose, but as yet Mark hasn't moved on from daily supervised consumption. This is therefore not likely to be a realistic option at this stage.

Mark was nodding. 'Yeah. I'll give him a call. Haven't spoken to Rod for a while, yeah, I'll see what he thinks. I mean, I've no reason to be around here, not really. Yeah, I've got some mates and, well, maybe they'll keep in touch if I moved permanently, but most of the people I know are from my drug days.'

'Mhmm. And your mum?'

'I think she'd be pleased to know I'm away. Things are easier but still difficult.'

The session continued with further thinking about getting away and what that would mean. Helen agreed to contact the local services once Mark could tell her where his cousin lived. He wasn't sure, just knew it was south west, somewhere in Devon, he thought.

Helen ended the session confirming the time they were meeting on Thursday. Mark again expressed appreciation that he was seeing her then, and she reminded him of the counselling on Wednesday.

Mark left feeling positive, the idea of heading south west for a few days and then, who knows, maybe more permanently, yeah, he could see that. Be near a beach, maybe get a job somewhere, bound to need people. Meet a few women as well, yeah, all that female flesh on the beaches in the summer. Yeah, he'd call Rod that evening, see what he had to say.

His cousin wasn't in; he left a message on his answerphone. Mark felt disappointed. He'd really geared himself up for that conversation. After he'd left the message he felt uncomfortable, kind of in limbo. Didn't know what to do with himself. He helped himself to a can of lager, seemed to take the edge off things a little, helped him relax. Well, the first one didn't, but by the third one, yeah, he was feeling quite chilled out.

Wednesday 5 July – counselling session
Tony, the counsellor, worked out of a small room in the clinic. It was also used by some of the other staff as well, for care co-ordination sessions when it was one-to-one. Fortunately, about six months before, there'd been a refurbishment and the room was now much more appropriate. Previously he had been using a room that was also an office for three of his colleagues. It was simply unsuitable but all that was available. Now that they had had the extension, there were two purpose-built rooms designated for client contact – not just for counselling, other members of the team also used them.

Tony went out to see if Mark had arrived. He had and he followed him down to the counselling room. Tony explained to Mark what counselling could offer and the limits to confidentiality. He explained that he had been given a summary of the situation – he wanted to be sure that Mark knew what he was aware of, enabling him to be open and authentic with his client. He told Mark how long he'd been working as a counsellor and how long he'd been at the community drug and alcohol service. He said that the sessions were 50 minutes and that while they did not have an upper limit to the number of sessions, generally they worked to about a year maximum. He indicated that this could be discussed at any time, that they would have review sessions although the review progress could take place at any time if Mark felt that would be helpful.

Mark listened. He was unsure quite what to expect. He'd been told by Helen that the counselling would be an opportunity to work therapeutically with emotional issues – and Mark knew he had some of those. He hadn't touched much on them with Helen; they had talked about more practical things, and the way he thought about his drug use. There had also been times when they'd looked at how he would cope up to the next session with her. Seemed to him that a lot of it was focused around his drug use and maybe he needed to talk more broadly. But that also felt rather unsettling. He didn't know what to say, so he sat and listened and waited.

'So, I'm interested in what you want to talk about, Mark. I don't want to direct you into any particular theme, rather I'd prefer to leave it for you to decide what you want to use this time to talk about, explore, make sense of, whatever emphasis you wish to place on it.'

Mark could feel his heart beating a little faster and he felt hot. He knew he wanted to talk about his past, his relationship with his mum, the feelings he felt about his life so far. So much was in his head but he sat, unable to say anything. Words going around in his head but none of them getting to his mouth.

'Can be difficult to start in – sometimes feelings get in the way.'

Mark nodded. 'Not sure what to say, really.'

'Not sure what to choose to say, where to start, lot to choose from?'

'Yeah, guess so. I mean, well, I mean you've read that summary and yeah . . .' Mark was thinking how weird it had been hearing himself described by someone he had never met. Felt kind of spooky, but he didn't say it. Didn't feel he could, somehow.

Tony nodded. 'Yeah, sounded like a difficult life so far for you.'

Mark snorted. 'Yeah, you could say that.' He shook his head. He didn't say any more. He didn't know what to say. Mark could feel himself sort of wanting to say things and in fact felt quite edgy about it. He kind of put that down to the fact that he hadn't had his methadone yet that day.

There was a lot of broken conversation and silence; it wasn't what Mark had expected. He'd kind of assumed there'd be lots of questions about his past, but no, this guy, Tony, seemed to just listen. Felt strange. Wasn't used to that. Didn't know quite what to do or say. People never listened to him; even as a child he'd never felt listened to. Just had to get on with it.

Although from the outside it might simply appear that there is a problem with communication, in reality therapy has started and Mark is experiencing his own expectations and beliefs about himself being confronted, simply because he is being listened to, and not being interrogated.

Mark had been sitting forward and he moved back in the chair. He wasn't sure why, just felt a bit stiff and wanted to relax a little.

Tony noticed it and considered that perhaps it was a sign that Mark at some level was relaxing a bit into the session. He also moved slightly in the chair, checking his own posture and noting that, yes, he'd been quite tense too. Often happened with a new client – natural human reaction.

'So, feeling a little more relaxed perhaps?'

Mark nodded. 'Still feels strange. What do you exactly do?'

Tony smiled warmly. 'I listen. I give people time, space to explore themselves. I endeavour not to judge anyone. I want to hear what people have to say, I want to appreciate and understand what's been going on for them, and what's happening now. But most of all it's a space, a free open space to reflect, review, to be. No agendas, no-one telling you what you should think or do, no-one on your case.'

'And that's it?'

'Mhmm. And it helps. That's my experience, and I hope that it helps you.'

'No-one's ever really listened, I mean, not until I started coming here. Helen listens. She encourages me, makes me think about things, makes me question what I'm doing. That's good. But you're not asking lots of questions.'

'I guess not. You expect questions, but I'm not giving them to you.'

'Feels strange. And I can talk about whatever I want?'

'Your agenda, your space, time for you.'

Mark was aware that his shoulders had tightened and he dropped them, deliberately, and took a deep breath. 'This is really different.'

'Yeah, it is, isn't it?' Tony didn't say any more, leaving it for Mark to explore the difference if he wanted to.

Mark smiled. 'And you just listen?'

'Mhmm. You feel like being listened to?'

'Shit, I don't know. I mean, I can usually talk, you know, no probs. But here, I don't know what to say.'

'Don't know what to say, or don't know what you want to have listened to?' Tony hadn't planned to say the second part; the words just flowed out from what he had already said.

'Guess I'm not sure that I feel OK about talking to you about some things.'

'Yeah, why should you feel good about me, you don't know me. Why should you tell me about things you've perhaps never told anyone else?'

Mark went quiet. 'I have to start talking to someone. I'll explode if I don't.'

'That's how it feels, like something in you is ready to explode, yeah?'

Mark took a deep breath and responded. 'Yeah. So much.' He shook his head. 'Just left to get on with my life, and I've fucked up, didn't think so at the time, but I have. Fucked up.'

'Life feels fucked up for you.'

'I feel fucked up.'

Tony nodded. 'Fucked up, that's how you feel.'

Mark could feel anger but not much else. No, there was another feeling but he didn't know what it was, just felt uncomfortable.

Tony recognised for himself that he didn't know exactly what Mark meant when he said 'fucked up', and he wanted to understand what it was that Mark experienced when he used those words.

'Not sure what you mean exactly, Mark, guess I'm aware of what "fucked up" means to me but not sure what it means for you.'

Bloody weird, thought Mark, fucked up means fucked up. 'Well,' his voice sounded irritated, 'you know, fucked up, does my head in.'

'Mhmm, does your head in. That's where you feel fucked up.' Tony raised his hand to his head.

'Yeah, well, no, I mean, shit I wish I could jack up. I just want to get away from stuff. Does my fucking head in.' Mark had put his head in his hands and had rubbed his eyes. He was suddenly feeling tired.

'Yeah, I hear you, Mark, it's just that I really want to understand what that means for you. Does your head in. Messes up your thinking?'

'Dunno, just leaves me sort of . . . well,' he paused, 'I don't know.' He rubbed his head in his right hand, causing his hair to stand up on end. He continued to rub it and then his forehead.

'Hard to say what it is but it leaves you rubbing your head. Frustrating, huh?'

Mark nodded. 'Yeah.' He took another deep breath and looked at the clock. Another 20 minutes or so to go. This wasn't what he expected. He thought it would be, well, he'd hoped it would be kind of easy, but this wasn't easy. Didn't feel easy at all.

Tony waited, maintaining his focus on Mark, holding his openness to what was present for him as he sat with Mark. While he felt comfortable he also felt this sense of pressure, like something wanted to break out or blow out. Over the years Tony had learned to trust these kinds of feelings. It just had a persistent presence.

'I don't know if this has meaning to you, but I'm sensing a kind of pressure, like something wants to blow out, maybe explode in some way.'

'I do. I want to blow it all away, blow it all out of my head. Start again. Blast it away, yeah. That would be good, blast all the shit out of my head.'

'Mhmm, that's what you want, to blast it all away, get shot of the shit, yeah?'

'And I'm fucking gonna do it, you know, I've got to. But I get confused, I want to get my arse into gear, and, yeah, Helen's good with that, you know. I've got to get a grip on my life.' Mark's right elbow was on the arms of the chairs and he sat holding his forehead in his hands, kneading his temples. He was feeling a head-ache coming on.

Mark found himself speaking. 'My childhood was pretty chaotic, you know. Mum sort of tried to bring us up – me and my brother – he's older than me and he left when he was 16, he had a tough time too and moved away from the area. He left just after my father went and mum started seeing this new guy, Eric. He didn't like us, but I was stuck. At least Trev got away. He had problems, but he's had therapy and seems to have helped him sort his head out. Married now, couple of kids and yeah, he's got it together. He gets depressed sometimes, but he's found a way out of it. But I got left, stuck with it all.' His jaw tightened. 'If dad hadn't pissed off, maybe it'd have been better, though he and mum argued a lot and it wasn't too good. But Eric, fuck's sake, creepy bastard. What my mum saw in him, God only knows. He stayed for a few years. Finally left but I was already into the gear, already fucked up by it all.' Mark was looking down and his hands were clenched.

'Really does get to you, thinking back to those times.'

'Fucking does. Bastard.'

'Eric?'

'Yeah, but I was thinking about dad. Went off with some other woman, saw him for a while after he left. He didn't go far, but I didn't like her. She wasn't interested in me either. Both parents shacked up with people who don't want to know you.' He shook his head.

'Hard to believe but it happened.'

Mark continued to shake his head. 'And, well, you know, kind of got into trouble, you know, at school, got excluded a few times and, well, ended up using. Tried different things at different times but really got into chasing, just got me out of it all. Fucking nightmare. Loved the feelings, the sensations. Yeah. Got me through it, but fucked me up as well.'

'So the effect of your parents' actions, the people they then had relationships with, school, chasing – it all adds up to a messed up childhood, yeah?'

'Yeah. And I can't seem to get it out of my head.'

'What do you mean exactly? Memories? Feelings? Thoughts?'

Mark shook his head. 'Dunno. Just don't feel right.'

'Don't feel right?' Tony's tone of voice invited Mark to say more.

'Just don't feel normal.' Mark was shaking his head. 'Huh. Don't know what normal is. Trev's got it together. I need to try and be like that as well, but, well, we don't really get on well now. He sort of gave up on me I guess with the smack, couldn't accept it I guess, and, well, I'd upset him a few times as well.'

'So it's not a good relationship then between you; he isn't someone you can turn to?'

'Nah. He's got his own life. I need to get mine together.' He paused. 'Talked to Helen about maybe going and seeing my cousin in Devon or somewhere, getting away for a bit.'

'Mhmm. That an idea that you're planning for?'

'Dunno. Tried calling last night but he wasn't there. Left a message. Maybe he'll call me tonight. He's my mother's older sister's son. Kind of get on well with him, you know? So, well, maybe. Dunno. Thought I'd just go down and see what it's like down there.'

The session continued with Mark exploring his thoughts about this idea.

As the session drew to a close, Tony drew Mark's attention to it and asked what he felt about the session and said that he felt good himself about working with Mark.

Mark said he'd like to come again, that it seemed difficult but now that they'd got into it, it seemed helpful somehow. Felt good to talk but felt strange to be really listened to. Said he'd have to think about that. Made him feel a bit weird, a good weird but strange nevertheless.

They agreed to weekly contact. Tony asked if there was anything specific Mark wanted to focus on, or did he want to take it session by session. Mark said he preferred the latter, though one of the things identified with Helen was his anger. Maybe he'd come back to that. Tony said that suited him, that he preferred to work that way, to flow more organically with what was present for the client. He commented that Mark was going through a lot of change, and different things could come up, and that in the final analysis he, Mark, knew what felt most pressing. The session ended.

Mark left feeling a little unsure what it was all about. Tony seemed to really take on board what he was saying. Funny, he was probably old enough to be his father, but it had begun to feel easy talking to him. It did feel odd but, yeah, it also felt important.

Tony sat back and reflected in the session, writing up his notes. He also dropped a line to Helen to say that Mark had attended and was engaging in the process, and that they would continue taking it one session at a time, building the therapeutic relationship and letting Mark set his own agenda for what he wanted to bring to the sessions.

Thursday 6 July – care co-ordination
'Seemed OK.' Mark was describing his impression of Tony to Helen at their session the next day.

'Mhmm. Good. Find it helpful?'

'Yeah, think so. Felt good talking but a bit strange. He really listens, doesn't he? I mean, you do too, but somehow he's different.'

'Yeah, well, he works differently. Therapeutic counselling isn't the same as care co-ordination and general support. But I'm glad you've made a start. It's early days, of course.'

'Yeah, well, we'll see how it goes.'

Mark went on to talk about the conversation he'd had the previous evening with Rod, who'd phoned him back. He'd been away, they'd been on holiday, but were back and, yeah, he'd be happy for Mark to come down for a few days, get a break from it all.

'I kind of explained about the help I was getting. He was really supportive. Also said I ought to tell Trev. He keeps in touch with him, and he thinks Trev'd be encouraging as well now that I'm doing something. Not sure about that, not yet. Maybe later. Anyway, yeah, he said I could come down, maybe over a weekend so as not to disrupt what I'm getting here. So I'm wondering about the weekend after next. Would that be possible?'

'OK, I'll need to contact the local service. How about if I do that now and see what's possible. I've had a chat with Dr Ashton and he's happy to give you a prescription for daily pick-up from a pharmacy down there. He figured that perhaps supervised consumption may not be necessary – you're out of area and, well, you'll only be dispensed one day's worth at a time.'

Mark explained where Rod lived and Helen checked through the list of local services, and phoned the local NHS Community Drug and Alcohol Service. They were really helpful, and said that while they did not yet have a pharmacist dispensing within their team – though this was planned and they were currently seeking funding for this – there were pharmacies close to where Rod lived, in fact one was actually in a parade of shops very close by, and they had a good relationship with them. They gave her the number of this, and a couple of alternatives who were also fairly close, so she could talk to them, check when they were open. Turned out they would be open, but not on the Sunday. They could give out two separate bottles for the Saturday and the Sunday though. Helen said she would need to check it with the prescribing doctor and would get back to them. She called the other two pharmacies and one was open for dispensing on the Sunday morning and, yes, they were used to supervising consumption.

She said they'd discuss it with Dr Ashton on Monday and that it would give them enough time to talk to the pharmacies.

Mark was OK with that, said he'd call Rod back that evening. Thought he'd maybe go down on the Thursday and come back Sunday. Wasn't too far for him to get down there, trains ran direct from where he lived. Then he'd be back for his script on the Monday. Said he'd be OK missing the session with her the next Thursday, but he'd have the counselling on the Wednesday.

Helen felt good that Mark was going away, would help to get him out and maybe his cousin would be a good influence on him. Sounded like he was really supportive. She wanted to be sure, however, that they'd got the prescribing clear. She knew from experience that the unexpected could happen.

Mark didn't mention the issue from the previous session regarding Stuey. Helen didn't raise it as it seemed Mark had other factors on his mind. She wanted to feel sure that Mark was confident about going to his cousin's. She felt a bit 'mothering' towards him. She didn't want this to turn out to be a bad experience. She wanted Mark to feel good about it, and then, well, maybe it would be the start of a fresh life.

Monday 10 July – prescribing clinic
At the session with Dr Ashton it was agreed to go for the pharmacy that was open, that he could take his methadone on the Thursday at the clinic and then head down to his cousin's, and that the pharmacy would be ready to receive his prescriptions for the Friday, Saturday and Sunday. Dr Ashton suggested that maybe they could think of switching his script to supervised consumption at one of the pharmacies that were closer to where he lived, if he felt OK about that. There were a couple that were happy supervising consumption. They'd review it when Mark got back.

Mark was happy with this. It wasn't always easy getting over to the clinic although in a way it did take up some of his day getting there. But it did mean he'd avoid a few people, and that felt good.

When he met up with Helen afterwards, he was telling her how much he was looking forward to getting away for a few days. 'It's only a couple of hours on the train, never thought of going down before, well, guess I was too out of it, too much to do, scoring and the like. At least the methadone is giving me an opportunity to get away.'

'Has some advantages then!'

'Yeah. Don't like it but I know I have to have it to keep myself together. Don't want to cut it back though, that'd be too much.'

'No, well, we're not there either. Let's get you really stable, get your life together and then, who knows, we always review things. You may change, you know? May want to get it out of your system. But that's ahead. Any urges to use on top this week?'

Mark shook his head. 'No. I felt good. You know, having something to look forward to, that feels really good. Yeah.'

'Mhmm. Makes a difference, yes?'

Mark nodded. 'Like I only ever really had scoring to look forward to, you know, took over, nothing else mattered, not really. But, yeah, managed to keep myself away from thinking about it.'

'Any time when you had to deliberately distract yourself?'

'Not really.'

'Not really?'

'Well, Saturday night was, well, Nick and Paula were out and, well, I find it hard on my own sometimes. Wondered about going out, but didn't feel like going to the pub. Not really a pub drinker, and, well, wondered who I could get in touch with, but everyone I thought about uses, you know. Felt depressed about that. Made me realise how much it had taken over my life. Made me sad.'

'And that sadness was difficult to handle?'

Mark nodded. 'Had a few lagers, that helped.'

'Often using the lager to deal with feelings?'

'A bit.'

'What's "a bit" mean, Mark?'

'Well, yeah, I did on Saturday, and yeah earlier in the week, when I'd tried to call Rod but he was out. That left me disappointed and I had a few lagers then as well.'

They discussed how Mark processed the feelings that left him wanting alcohol. It was clear that Mark had a low tolerance of feelings, particularly those that he defined as uncomfortable.

'How about after the counselling?'

'No. But then I felt more weird than uncomfortable. I mean, I got back and Paula was there and I had a chat with her. Yeah, had a can, but just the one. Didn't really feel I needed it.'

'Strong lager?'

'No, around 5%. Just relaxed with it and then Nick came in. Yeah. Felt OK about the counselling. It was the other times.'

'Guess I'm aware that both could have left you disappointed – I mean, people not being there, you know, Nick and Paula out, Rod not there to answer the phone.'

'People not being there for me – yeah, there's a theme all right. Goes back a long, long way that one.'

'Sensitive area I guess. And I guess it's about how you think about the feeling. You plan something, or have an expectation, but it doesn't work out how you planned.'

'Yeah, I thought Nick and Paula were going to be in, but they weren't. They said they'd told me, guess I'd forgotten. But yeah, you plan something and then it doesn't happen. Don't like that.'

'So how do you feel, other than disappointed?'

Mark thought about it. 'Well, frustrated I guess, kind of irritated.'

'And I guess I'm wondering if these are the feelings you drink on or to get away from?'

'Probably. Just pisses me off, you know, and yeah, then I grab a can or two.'

'So something doesn't happen the way you plan or expect it, you get disappointed first, and then frustrated and irritated?'

'Guess so.'

'Then you drink.'

Mark nodded.

'So these kinds of feelings are drinking triggers, sort of put you at risk, yeah?'

'Yeah.'

'So, we need to look at ways of managing these feelings. Tony'll be more interested in helping you resolve the experiences that make you sensitive to them in the way that you are.'

'Don't know about managing them.'

'Not something you've kind of had to think about.'

'Well, no, I mean, I guess I've just avoided feelings, you know?'

'Mhmm.'

'And now I'm not on the smack, well, sometimes ... it's difficult. Sometimes I just wish I'd wake up and it would all be OK.' Mark sighed heavily.

Helen followed it up. 'What would that ideal world be like, Mark?'

'Hassle-free. Doing what I want, be settled down. Yeah, steady job, I guess, and getting on with my life. No mess in my head, just, well, normal, 'cept I'm not sure what normal is.'

'So you'd like something more "normal" and that involves a steady job, feeling settled, no mess in your head, and just getting on with life, with doing what you want.'

Mark listened to what he had been saying being repeated back. Yeah. That was what he wanted, but he had to get his head straight, he knew that. Had to sort out his past. 'Yeah, have to sort out the past, don't I, get a grip on it all, give myself a chance.'

'A chance . . .?'

'Of a fresh start. Yeah, I want to leave the past behind, but I can't, it's fucked me up and now, well, now I'm stuck with it.'

Helen nodded. She saw many clients whose upbringing was chaotic, unpredictable, uncertain. She knew that these were factors that contributed to problems in adult life (Velleman, 2001).

'Yeah, must feel like you've got it for life, and yet people can change, redefine themselves, learn new reactions and behaviours.'

'You think so?' Mark was looking straight into Helen's eyes.

'Oh yes, we can learn new ways of being, new ways of coping with life. You're learning to cope without the smack, and now it's about learning to cope without so much alcohol and perhaps, in the future, it'll be about learning to cope without the methadone, but we take it slowly, no rush, change has to be sustainable, yeah? We need you off the alcohol as much as possible and stable on the methadone.'

'Sounds like a lot to deal with.'

'It is, that's why it's got to be slowly, slowly, yeah? No pushing, but maybe a few gentle nudges, and if something happens that triggers you into using or drinking, well, we sit down, look at it, make sense of it, give you a chance to explore what you feel about it, and then try and learn from it.'

Mark nodded. 'Yeah.'

'So with the alcohol there's frustration and irritation, and they both follow on from feeling disappointment when something doesn't work out as you had planned it or anticipated it.'

Helen brings the focus back to the cognitive-behavioural theme that had emerged earlier in the session. As the care co-ordinator she will be wanting to ensure that the risk of relapse is minimised and that Mark develops strategies to cope with risky situations. She is not offering therapeutic counselling, and she is being directive, seeking to work with the theme that emerged earlier and which was not fully resolved.

'Yeah. Guess I find it hard when I don't get my way. Sounds a bit childish.'

'Remind you of being a child, or just seems childish?'

'Never got my own way much, well, I suppose I did in that I was often left to get on with things, and that was OK, but it wasn't as well. I mean, I'd have liked a different life at home and I didn't get that. I could go out and about pretty much as I pleased, mum didn't seem too bothered, but then, sometimes, she'd go ballistic. Now I know it was the drugs, she'd get all wound up – clucking maybe, I don't know – and I'd do something and she'd flare up at me.'

'Happened a lot?'

Mark nodded. He could remember it as if it was yesterday, some of it anyway. He could remember coming in one day from school; he'd had a bad time getting hassle from other kids. Came in, put his music on real loud. His mum had burst into the room, hauled the plug out and started screaming at him. He'd felt terrified, she'd really lost it. Told him he was grounded – he never was, she'd forget, or get too out of it to care – and then she stormed out of the room. Nothing more had happened but he remembered, vividly, her standing there screaming at him, telling him he was a selfish little shit, she was trying to sleep, never got a moment's peace, telling him he was no good. As he recalled the event he felt a surge of emotion, remembering one sentence very clearly. 'Told me she wished she'd never had me. I'll never forget that.'

Helen realised that this was another therapy issue that could more usefully be dealt with by the counsellor; she wasn't clear as to how much of a traumatic effect it must have had on Mark, and what other traumas remained undisclosed that may be deeper – known or forgotten.

'Something not easy to forget.'

'I never will. I guess something changed for me then. I knew that I was kind of on my own. I mean, I'd tried to be what she wanted, tried to keep out of sight and stuff, but I guess from then on I just didn't care any more.'

'So something shifted, changed.' Helen was aware that they were sliding towards therapy and once again away from the focus on managing irritation. And yet ... It was all linked up. She stayed with Mark, trusting the wisdom of his need to voice what was present for him.

'Didn't care much after that. Didn't care about her, or her boyfriend. Just got on with my life. And got into trouble, more and more.'

'Must have been frustrating?'

'S'pose so, but, well ...' He went quiet. Mark was aware that he was suddenly feeling a lot more than he had before.

Helen kept her attention on Mark. Mark felt distinctly uncomfortable and forced himself away from the feelings that were around for him. He didn't want to go there. He looked up at the clock; time was nearly up.

'I'd better head off. Not feeling too good. Feeling tired.' He yawned.

Helen was aware of feeling frustrated herself, that Mark seemed to be heading off and, to her, avoiding this theme of disappointment, frustration and irritation. She was aware that she was feeling those things herself. She decided to voice them, thinking it might be useful for Mark to know that she also experienced these kind of feelings. Sort of make the relationship more even, but she didn't want to be judgemental though the truth was that was how she felt.

'I'm aware of feeling disappointed, in fact, all the feelings that we've highlighted – irritation, frustration – as I was anticipating we'd spend more time focusing on them. And I appreciate that you want to leave, but I just wanted to use this as an example of what can cause these feelings to arise.'

Mark shrugged. 'I'm tired. I need to go.'

Helen was concerned – they hadn't talked much about the trip south west. 'And you're OK for Devon, yeah?'

'Got my script, yeah, and I'll see how it goes.'

Helen was very aware that he had taken the focus away and that he wasn't coming across as someone who was comfortable with himself. Was it wise for him to go away? Had he touched something deep and difficult and was that going to put him at risk? Helen was uncertain. She decided the best response was to make visible her concerns, acknowledging what she sensed to be happening but not dwelling on it. Letting Mark know what had become present for her.

'I'm just aware that you changed the focus and wanted to end the session quickly, though, yes, time is nearly up. But my concern is whether what we talked about today has touched something deep for you and it's making it all that much more difficult. I mean, what I'm saying is, I want you to ...' Helen was aware that she was rambling but she had to end the sentence. 'Take care of yourself, Mark, I really hope the weekend goes well and I'll see you next week.'

'Thanks. Yeah. I'll be fine. See you.'

Mark headed off. He still felt troubled but he didn't want to let Helen know. He didn't want to talk about it. He dropped off at the off-licence on the way home for a few lagers. He felt better after he'd drunk them – well, different.

Wednesday 12 July – counselling session
Ten minutes had passed since the time Mark's counselling session should have started, but Mark had not appeared. No sign of him. No message from him during the day. Tony wondered what might have happened. Had he decided not to come? He continued to wait.

Mark hadn't been into the clinic earlier in the day for his methadone. He'd over-slept, then he wasn't sure that he wanted to go in, knew the counsellor was there and he wasn't sure he wanted to talk to Tony. Got it in his head that Tony would make him feel bad, make him relive stuff from the past. Truth was he didn't want to feel, to feel what had become present for him with Helen. He'd drunk too much lager, had fallen asleep in the early hours and had woken up feeling really groggy. He'd felt worse as the day went on, aware that he needed his methadone. He knew he wanted to use, so many of his plans were fading, just the thought of using, the thought of that lovely silky feeling, of floating away from everything, everything. Oh yeah, that was what he needed.

Summary

Mark acknowledges his need for change, and the idea of moving out of area comes to him. He starts to investigate this. Mark has his first counselling session – he finds it hard adjusting to it, but begins to talk about his past. He discusses further the idea of moving away and a suitable pharmacy is found for supervised consumption. Dr Ashton agrees to this. Mark has a heavy drinking session and doesn't make it to the next counselling session. The feelings of using have become strong once again.

CHAPTER 6

Using on top, and a way ahead emerges

- Methadone maintenance (Tier 3)
- Care co-ordination (Tier 3)
- Structured therapeutic counselling (Tier 3)
- Day programme waiting list (Tier 2)

Thursday 13 July

It was mid-afternoon and Mark hadn't come in for his methadone. Tony had left a message for Helen which she picked up when she got back from a couple of home visits. Damn, she thought, what's going on. She called the number for Paula and Nick. There was no answer. She left a message on the answerphone. Paula and Nick knew the situation so she didn't feel she was breaching confidentiality. She was concerned. She wanted to check that Mark was OK ... She knew he was only scripted for Friday to Sunday. He wouldn't be able to just stop. Something must have gone wrong. She left it for an hour and called again. Still no answer. Shit, she thought. At least she knew that his scripts were for daily doses; he wasn't going to be out there with a large bottle of methadone, and at risk of overdosing.

The initial confidentiality agreement with Mark made it clear that Helen could call Nick and Paula. They were aware of the situation. It is important to have someone that a service can contact if need be, particularly where a client is being prescribed and there is uncertainty as to what is happening. At least, because consumption is supervised, there is containment of that aspect; there is not the risk of Mark selling it on. But when Mark doesn't turn up for the methadone – and he would need something to stave off withdrawal – then there is a need to try to contact him or at least find out what has happened in the hope of reassuring him and bringing him back into the service for support and to review what can best be offered to minimise risk.

She tried calling again later in the afternoon, just before she headed home: still no reply. She left a message for the duty person the following morning to call her if Mark came in for his supervised consumption. She rather felt it unlikely, but, well, maybe he'd be back in touch. She also alerted Dr Ashton as to what had happened. They wondered about contacting the pharmacy in Devon, but that might just force Mark to use off the streets if they refused, and might mess up the opportunity for support from his cousin. They wanted to keep in contact with Mark, not threaten him and lose touch. They recognised the importance of harm minimisation. They could only wait, and keep trying to contact Nick and Paula.

Friday 14 July
The next morning there had been a phone message from Mark for Helen. He was sounding very distressed, must have called in the night. Said he was sorry, he'd used, he wanted to stop again, hadn't injected since the evening and was feeling rough. Wanted to come in first thing.

The message was relayed to Helen who came into the clinic. She called Mark as she had other appointments later in the morning and wanted to encourage him to come in while she was there. Paula answered, and passed the phone on to Mark. He was awake and feeling very shaky, but wanted to come in. He arrived 45 minutes later. Helen didn't have long to spend with him, but she'd spoken to her team leader about the situation who was in that morning and agreed to spend more time with Mark if he needed it.

Mark arrived; he'd actually tidied himself up a bit. He followed Helen into the counselling room.

'Sorry, I fucked up.'

'What happened?'

'Think I got into some heavy stuff last time I saw you, got to me more than I thought. Had a few drinks and, I dunno, started thinking crazy thoughts I guess. Decided I didn't want the counselling, that I'd be made to feel worse, you know, and I couldn't face it. And the more I thought about it, the worse it got.'

'Got out of control, your thoughts, yeah?'

Mark sighed. 'I'm really sorry. I know it was my head, but I just needed to get away from it and, well, I went out and scored, a few times. Couldn't hold it together. Then realised what an idiot I was, how much I was putting at risk, how you're all trying to help me. So I didn't use again from yesterday evening, but drank strong lager, got me through the night. Wasn't good. Phoned and, yeah, now I don't know.'

'So, yeah, scored a few times but then realised it was messing things up. So, where do we go from here?'

Mark was shaking his head. 'I don't know. I guess I've got to try again, you know, get back to the methadone. I'd been OK, but what we talked about, you know, feelings and stuff. Got to me. Really didn't think it had but, just had to use.'

'So you scored pretty soon after you saw me?'

'No, drank heavily, but it was the next day, just kept thinking about how the counselling was going to make me feel. Did my head in. Had to get away from it.

Knew the methadone wouldn't do it. Had to score. Used on Tuesday and into Wednesday. Madness.'

'So, two days of using, but nothing else, other than alcohol?'

Mark nodded.

'Clean needles?'

'Yeah. Had some stashed at home. Thank God for that. I really think I would have used dirty needles, I was just so all over the place.'

'Good. At least you haven't put yourself more at risk.'

'No. Anyway. I stayed away from Paula and Nick Tuesday night, came back late Wednesday. Told them what had happened. They were good, once they'd finished telling me what an idiot I was.'

'So, your plans now?'

'I still want to get away, get down to my cousin. I need a break, a change of scene. Need to get my head straight.'

'Think you're well enough to travel?'

Mark nodded. 'Yeah, I have to be. I'm feeling shaky but the meth will stop that.'

'OK, but I think you should stay here for a while, be sure you're OK before you head off.' Helen noticed the time. 'Look, I've got to head off. Jim, one of my colleagues, is around and he'll stay with you for a while and have a chat, and sort out the methadone for you. We've got it ready.'

'Thanks.'

'And you're sure you haven't used since yesterday? Don't want you overdosing.'

'No, honest, not since yesterday evening. 7.00pm.'

'How much?'

'Not a lot, I mean, really, not a lot, only had a little left.'

'OK.' She went out and found Jim who came in.

'Hi, Mark. Things been a bit messy, yeah? I'm sure it'll settle back down.'

'Yeah. Can I have the meth now?'

'Yeah, OK.' Jim glanced across to Helen.

'Yeah, that's fine, but stay around a while, yeah? And we'll talk about it more on Monday. Maybe we need to think again about what's going to help you be stable. Obviously there are things that upset you, make it difficult and, well, we need to think it through, yeah? See you Monday, we'll talk it through then.'

'OK. Thanks. And I'm really sorry. And can you let Tony know?'

'I can do. He said he can see you same time, same day next week. Perhaps you might want to leave him a note?'

'Yeah, yeah, that'd be good.' After Helen had gone Mark asked Jim for some paper and a pen. He scribbled a note to Tony, saying he was sorry he'd not come in, and he'd see him next week at the same time and hoped that this was OK.

Mark stayed for about 45 minutes, chatting to Jim about different things. He could feel the methadone kicking in, taking the edge off things. He began to feel easier in himself. Eventually he headed off, back home to get his stuff and then on to the station. He was glad things had been OK at the clinic. He really wasn't sure how they'd react. Thought they might have stopped prescribing, or taken his scripts away. But they hadn't, and he was grateful. He didn't feel worthy of being trusted after what had happened yet he felt good that they were trusting him, and not making it difficult or awkward. They seemed to appreciate the difficulty. He hadn't had a chance to say much to Helen, but he had spoken to Jim, who seemed a nice enough guy.

As he sat on the train he could still feel that pull to use, it was around – had been since Monday. He didn't like it. He wanted to feel in control. The next thing he knew was feeling the train jolt. He'd fallen asleep and it had just pulled in to his station. Shit, he thought as he grabbed his bag, and stumbled along the corridor and off the train. Rod had said he'd come and pick him up – he'd said he was going to be a bit later and it was nearly 1 o'clock. He saw him by the barrier. He looked good. Yeah, it was good to get away. But he was anxious, strangely anxious. Maybe this trip south west was more important to him than he realised. He knew he didn't want to fuck up again.

Monday 17 July – prescribing clinic
Mark had arrived early for his appointment with Dr Ashton. He was feeling good; the weekend had gone well after all. He saw Helen come down the corridor.

'Hi, Mark, come on through.'

He got up and followed her towards the consulting room, and turned in.

'Hi, Mark, how's it going?'

'OK. Yeah.' He thought about last week, and wasn't too sure how the doc was going to react. He had used on top, and he was supposed to be trying not to. 'Look, sorry, 'bout last week. It was stupid. Won't happen again.'

'It's not good using like this, Mark, but at least you're using mainly instead and not on top of the methadone. But you know the risks, you know the risk of overdose maybe, or it all just getting out of control.'

'Yeah, I know. And, well, I know it's me, finding it hard to handle stuff, yeah?'

'Not an easy time, I know.' Dr Ashton went on to check out what had happened, whether he'd used again since last Thursday. Mark said no, he'd stayed with the script and it had been OK at the pharmacy. Explained that it was stuff that had come up, feelings that, well, he wasn't too good with feelings. Dr Ashton empathised with his struggle. 'Yes, when you've had years keeping away from them they can be a shock.'

'Tell me about it.'

Dr Ashton wanted to know if Mark felt OK with their approach of trying to stabilise him on methadone, that there were other options: other medications he could prescribe, or detoxification. Mark shook his head. 'Can't see myself clean, don't want to be, not yet anyway. No. But the daily pick-up and having to drink it here, it's a pain, but I guess you're not gonna change that after last week?'

'No, we really need you to get stable, and we're hoping the counselling and the day programme will help you come to terms with maintaining your current script, and understand what tempts you into using and how that can be handled.'

'Yeah. I do want to be in control, I really do.' He was thinking back to the weekend. 'Had a good time away. I really could go down there, you know?'

'Where exactly?'

'North Devon coast. Know it?'

Dr Ashton nodded. 'Driven along it. So I guess you'll want to talk it through with Helen?'

'Yeah.'

'OK. So, we keep you on the same dose for now. We'll keep it under review though, and if you get stable, well, we can look at changing the prescribing, but we need the supervised consumption for now, Mark. But it won't be forever. You've just got to get it together.'

Mark nodded. 'Thanks. Yeah, I know.' He got up and left the room. Helen followed him out and into the counselling room for their care co-ordination session.

Is Dr Ashton too lenient with his prescribing, or is he being realistic? Should he insist on increasing the methadone to see if Mark is more stable? But is that the way to handle feelings that are more present for Mark? The methadone is to substitute for the heroin, not to provide emotional tranquillisation. If prescribed other tranquillisers, that would complicate the cocktail of substances, particularly with Mark using alcohol as well. While it may be a rollercoaster, at least Mark is now becoming more aware of his need for change, and if the chaos can be ridden through and support and encouragement maintained, then there is opportunity for Mark to move on. It can be a stressful time not only for clients, but also for the professionals. The need for appropriate levels of professional and personal support among people working in the drug and alcohol field is high. The client group is risky; there can a be a very thin line between life and death for the chaotic substance user.

Helen encouraged Mark to talk more about the weekend and about the problems from the previous week. Mark explained that he was still concerned about how strongly he had felt things after he'd seen her the previous Monday, and was concerned whether the counselling session would stir it all up.

'Do you think the counselling is happening too soon, that you maybe need something else?' Like more methadone, she thought to herself. She voiced her thoughts after a moment's hesitation.

'No, I mean, it wasn't the counselling that set me off, it was what came up here last week with you, and then my crazy head about what I thought would happen with Tony. No, I've got to persevere. I'm not wanting to mess you about, I am serious, but fuck it was crazy last week. Just had to use, get that feeling and get away. More methadone might damp things down, yeah, but that's what I want to get away from. I don't want it to go up, I'd only have to struggle to bring it back down again. No. I need to hold it together as I am.'

Helen smiled and nodded. 'Just aware of thinking that you did get away in another way as well last week and got a good experience out of it. There are other ways . . .'

'Not the same though.'

'No, don't suppose a weekend in North Devon is like a heroin rush. But that's the choice, isn't it?'

Mark nodded. Yeah, he thought, that's it exactly. He had to put it behind him, try again.

Helen continued. 'And I guess I'm wondering what the advantages of change are for you?' She suggested a life line to help him appreciate what the choice was about for him. She drew a line with a fork. The fork represented the point of choice, of decision. The lower fork was a continuation of the line, the other branched upwards (Bryant-Jefferies, 2001, p. 109).

'So, the lower is go back to using, don't change; the upper line is change. What are the positives of change?'

Mark thought about it. 'Feeling better, eventually. Not so likely to harm myself. Maybe get a different life, job, relationship, kids – is that a positive? Yeah, that'd be good, one day.' He paused and snorted. 'Yeah, feel normal, whatever that is.'

'OK.' Helen drew branches off the top of the higher line and wrote the different positives that Mark had identified. 'And what are the negatives of change, there will be some, things you'll miss, maybe?'

'Depends I guess. I mean, if I move I'll lose friends.'

'Friends, such as?'

Mark mentioned a few names, then hesitated. 'No, Nick and Paula are my real friends. All the others are using. I've got to leave them behind, haven't I?'

'Yeah, so is that a positive or negative?'

'I'd kind of miss them, but then, maybe I wouldn't.'

'Did you think of them much at the weekend?'

Mark shook his head. 'No.'

'So maybe you wouldn't if you moved away?'

Mark nodded. 'Yeah, maybe.'

'So you may miss friends, maybe not, but you'd miss not seeing so much of Nick and Paula?'

'Yeah. But then I guess a positive is that maybe I'd make new friends, and a few that are a bit more healthy for me too!'

'Yeah, very possible. OK, so "new friends" is a positive. Any other negatives from not using?'

Mark took a deep breath and let the air out slowly. 'No rush.' He spoke quietly.

'Not easy to say, huh?'

Mark shook his head. 'No, that's the big one.'

'Not getting that feeling.'

'That feels like the really big one, Helen, still can't really imagine it.'

'Too close, too vivid?'

Mark nodded. Yeah, he thought, shit, never use again, *never* seemed a bloody long time. 'I can't see it. I want to, but I can't, Helen, I hate the stuff but I fucking love it as well.' He closed his eyes. 'Shit, it's so fucking hard. I mean, last week, Christ I had to score, Helen, I had to. I didn't have a choice. I *had* to.'

She nodded. 'Yeah, it's still all so close, so alive to you, and, yeah, easy to get – you know who's dealing, it's easy.'

'Too fucking easy. Wish I could forget who bloody well deals. Wish some-one could hypnotise me, make me forget about it, take away the memory and let me get on with my life,' he paused, 'and I'd hate that too, the thought of not remembering, or not being able to recall the feelings, the sensations.' As he spoke, Mark could feel himself drifting into happy memories.

'Compelling, yeah?'

Mark didn't reply straight away; he'd heard Helen but she seemed distant . . .

Helen waited for a few seconds before responding. 'You seem to have drifted off, Mark.'

'Hmm, yeah, sorry.' He smiled grimly. 'Can't get it out of my head. It's gonna take a while, isn't it?'

'Probably. Takes time to bring it under control and recover from the kind of chaotic use you've had in the past.'

'Yeah, I know.' He paused again, but this time held his focus. 'Oh, I forgot to say, I've an appointment with the other service about the day programme. Seeing them on Friday, just for a kind of chat, to get to know me and for me to get to know them.'

'That's great. So things are coming together.'

Mark nodded. 'Just got to make the most of it. I am determined, Helen, it's just that . . .'

'Just that . . .?'

'I just can't see myself drug-free and stable, and normal and stuff. Can't see it.'

Helen glanced at the clock – they had another 20 minutes. She picked up the life line they'd been drawing. 'Yeah, the things you have here – getting a job, relationship, feeling normal, kids – but it's hard to imagine them.'

'It is.'

'Shall we continue with the life line, or do you want to focus on this struggle to really imagine what life would be like.'

'Let's finish it.'

'OK. We've got the positives and negatives of change. What are the positives and negatives of not changing? Positives first.'

'The whole experience, scoring, habit, not having to think about things too much.'

'OK, so scoring, the whole habit, the effect it has on, what, feeling responsible?'

'Nothing to feel responsible about, really, just drift along. I'm used to it, you know?'

'And it's a positive experience for you, being like this?'

Mark was about to say yes, but it didn't feel right. 'Sort of but no as well. I mean, yeah,' he shrugged his shoulders, 'but it's messing me up. But I'd miss it.'

'Yeah, you'd miss it but it messes you up. It would be good to carry on as you have been, but it messes you up as well.'

'Fed up being messed up.'

'Yeah, being messed up doesn't have much going for it, yeah?'

'Does my head in. It was kind of easier when I was using, I mean, I could control my head more? Now, well, it's not so easy.'

Helen nodded. 'Yeah, that feeling of being messed up in your head, would be good to get away from it, but it may help short term, but beyond that . . .'

'. . . fucks me up.' Mark screwed his eyes up and rubbed his forehead and his eyes. He then slammed his fist down on the arm of the chair. 'Fuck it. I have to kick it, fucking have to, fucking hate it, hate it. I feel all over the fucking place sometimes.'

'Only sometimes. I'm wondering what enables you to not feel like it all of the time?'

'The methadone helps, it really does. Takes the edge off things a lot, but not always. Being with Nick and Paula, that sometimes helps. My music, that's important to me.'

'So, things that kind of distract you, or give you something to focus on?'

Mark nodded.

'I'm wondering then what else might be added to this to help you get your focus and feel a bit away from feeling messed up in your head.'

'Alcohol helps.' He smiled. 'It's true, no point in denying it.'

'Yeah. You're right. It plays a part.'

'A big part.'

'Mhmm. Feel OK about that?'

'No. It's not the answer, but it helps. It's hard to not use something that makes you feel better.'

'That's the problem, isn't it, hard not to use something when you know it'll make you feel a little easier.'

'You think this day programme'll work?'

'I'm sure it will help you, Mark. It'll help you make sense of yourself, give you strategies to cope with situations and thoughts. And you'll learn from other participants – bound to.'

'You sound very positive about it.'

'Sounds like you're not.'

'I dunno.'

Helen was aware of the ambivalence and the contradictions in what Mark was saying. 'So you're determined to get in control, want to take the help that's offered, but you're kind of not convinced it'll work?'

'Well, it doesn't always, does it?'

'No. But that's other people. We're talking about you and working in ways to make sure that it works for you.'

Mark rubbed his nose. 'Guess I want too much too soon. Want it all to be better.'

'Quick fix, huh? Magic wand?'

'It's not like that, is it?'

Helen shook her head. 'You're accustomed to quick fixes, Mark, it's probably hard for you to tolerate anything that takes time, but that's part of the process of recovery – learning to tolerate a longer process, learning to step back from that urge to get things sorted immediately, to get relief from feeling bad instantly.'

Mark looked across at the life line. 'Yeah, that's another positive of not changing; instant is better than long-winded.'

'Yeah, you'd rather have the quick fixes? You're going to miss them.'

Mark nodded. 'And I know that's part of the habit, part of the nightmare.' He cupped his chin in his hand and shook his head. 'But that line for not changing, you know, you've drawn it as a shorter line.'

Helen nodded. Yes, she had, deliberately, to have the opportunity of highlighting another factor although some people might regard it as positive rather than negative – a shorter life. 'Mhmm.'

'Hmmm.' Mark tightened his lips. 'Yeah,' he sighed, 'and that's the bottom line, isn't it?'

Helen nodded, not wanting to say anything to detract from Mark's experience of what he was processing as he considered the implications of the shorter line. 'Yeah, I don't want a shorter line. Quick fix can mean a quick life.' He shook his head. 'I want something more, I want something better. I really do.' He paused again. 'I need a fresh start, I'm beginning to realise that more and more. I need a new environment, but I need to get my head straight otherwise I'm just going to carry on as I have, aren't I?'

'That's the risk. That is the risk.'

'Yeah. OK. Yeah. And, well, I can keep in touch with Nick and Paula, but I know when I was away, you know, I was feeling different. I was less uptight, just seemed to be able to chill a bit. Felt good. I need to get myself together, get used to what I'm being offered here and then move on. Though I'm also wondering whether I ought to move away now and do all this somewhere else. What do you think?'

Helen thought about it and was so aware that she could see pros and cons with either choice. In truth, she didn't know. 'I really don't know. I'm aware that we haven't got much more time today; is that something you want to think about? I mean, consider the life line we've been doing today; how about doing another specifically around the idea of whether you move away now, or not? One line to represent staying here, one to represent moving away?'

Mark nodded; that sounded like a good idea. He didn't know either. He felt he was leaning more towards getting away, but he was getting good support, he liked Helen and Dr Ashton, and he was getting to know Tony and he knew the clinic and was familiar with a number of the staff. The thought of starting over felt uneasy, and yet ... 'Seems like a good idea. I'll do that. I don't know either, but maybe it'll give us something to think about next time.'

'Mmm. And, you know, just be aware that they'll be similar services where you are going, you know, that's one of the things that is changing these days, so, you know, bear that in mind.'

'OK.'

One key feature of the current changes in drug services is that of ensuring that services across the country are brought into line with similar standards and services on offer. Of course, there will always be local variation in order to ensure services are appropriate and responsive to local needs, but people requiring services should have access to a basic range of services throughout the country. For Mark at this stage that means a prescribing clinic with supervised consumption of methadone, care co-ordination, therapeutic counselling and a day programme.

The session drew to a close with agreement about the next appointment on Thursday.

Wednesday 19 July – counselling session
The following counselling session involved Mark starting by apologising again, and saying why he hadn't come along, the ideas in his head, why he was thinking them as a result of that earlier care co-ordination session with Helen. In fact, it didn't leave him feeling how he had expected and it led him into talking more about his childhood experiences and how he felt towards what had happened. It included a lot of 'story telling'. Somehow Mark was experiencing a sense of a need to describe how it was, and it felt good that Tony listened. Tony didn't have to say a great deal, clarifying a few points as the story unfolded.

Mark spoke about the incident when his mum had told him she wished she hadn't had him, which had made him shy away from the last counselling session. Mark felt awful as he spoke, all kinds of sensations inside him. Tony was very gentle, not pushing him in any way, maintaining a classical person-centred approach, staying with Mark, being a sensitive companion as Mark revealed more and more of his inner world. Tony was aware that there were now 15 minutes left of the session and he was aware of his own anxiety as to how Mark would feel when he left the session. While he instinctively felt trust towards Mark, and to the process of change and development that was occurring within him, he well recognised that medication and other drugs could disrupt this, leaving the client maybe more at risk of an attitude of mind and a resulting set of behaviours that could cause risk to themselves. He voiced the time, and highlighted his concern as to the impact the theme that had developed in the counselling would have on Mark.

'Actually, I feel a bit of relief. I feel weird as well, all these strange feelings, but I've got to learn to face it, haven't I? And I'm getting so much support to achieve this. And once the day programme starts, well, I guess I'll be seeing some each day for a while, and that'll be good.' He also then mentioned the work he was doing with Helen about whether to move away or not, and Tony empathised with the dilemma.

'Is that something you want to talk about here, or keep the discussions with Helen?'

'I want to keep them with Helen. I feel I need to use this time to make sense of myself, of my past. That's what seems most important.'

'Fine. So you're feeling a bit of relief but aware of feeling weird as well.'

Mark nodded. He looked out of the window. It sort of struck him that there was a world out there that he wasn't part of. The thought struck him quite forcibly. Something he already knew, but somehow it suddenly felt more real, more present.

Tony watched him and wondered what had caught his eye. He waited for a moment then glanced out of the window himself.

Mark sensed him doing this. It brought his own attention back into the room. 'Drifted off a bit there.'

'Mhmm. Something catch your eye?'

'No, a thought, how I'm missing out on what's going on out there, and I need to get into a new life, a life I've never really had.'

'Yeah. New life, and for you it'll be really new, yeah?'

Mark nodded. Yeah, he thought, that really was it. Really new. That left him feeling uneasy. He knew what he was used to. Could he do it? He knew he had to. He'd done the stuff Helen had suggested and he was coming round to realising that he wanted to move on, move down to the south west, start again, new surroundings, new people, but he wanted to be sure about the support he'd receive. He'd decided to raise this with Helen on Thursday.

Mark mentioned what he was thinking about, said he hadn't made a final decision, but he was giving it serious thought.

Tony felt disappointed, he felt that he was experiencing a rapport with Mark and, yeah, he cared about him and wanted him to move away from the lifestyle that had been his for so many years. Yeah, he liked to think he could play a part in helping Mark towards a healthier future, towards perhaps a more authentic sense of self. 'Well, if you stay, I really hope I can help you towards the new life that you want, and if you go, yeah, I'll miss you, and I know there are others who work as I do and I'm sure they'll give you the same kind of help.'

They moved into discussing how Mark was going to deal with the feelings that were still present for him. 'Kind of feel I need a drink, but that's not what I'm going to do. In a way feels more difficult to plan what to do because I'm not sure if I'm going to stay here.'

'Sort of in limbo, yeah?'

Mark nodded. 'Yeah, but I have to get down to it. Think I'll head back home, maybe go and see my mum. Things are a little better with her. See how it goes.' The session drew to a close and Mark left. Tony was aware of how much more Mark was getting in touch with his childhood, with his feelings towards his mother. Wasn't sure quite how Mark would be seeing his mother after having had the session, but that was Mark's choice. He felt sure that he had every reason for this.

Thursday 20 July – care co-ordination

'I don't know, Helen, I really don't know.'

Mark was sitting in the counselling room with Helen. It was pouring with rain outside, and he'd drunk too much the night before. He hadn't intended to, and it wasn't the result of the session with Tony, he knew that. It was his mum. It was after he'd seen her.

'What's happening?' Helen deliberately said 'happening' rather than 'happened', to keep the focus in the present.

'I felt I'd made a decision, you know, and now, I dunno.'

'So you're unsure again?'

Mark nodded. 'I did a life line, haven't brought it with me, doesn't seem much point at the moment.'

Helen stayed silent, keeping her attention on Mark. He continued.

'I went to see my mum after the session with Tony yesterday. I don't know, we started arguing again, and I told her I was going to leave, go and stay with Rod, get away from everything. She just fell apart, got all emotional, told me I couldn't go, she needed me, couldn't bear me being away. It just got out of control. I was confused. I wanted to go, then I didn't. I wanted to tell her to fuck off, but I couldn't. I just, I don't know, just . . .' He shrugged his shoulders.

'Lost it?'

'I mean, I'm hardly there, I thought she'd encourage me, be glad I was doing something, or at least be glad to see the back of me for a while. But no, she started going on about how hard it would be for her to cope, how worried she'd be.' Mark was shaking his head. 'Never seemed that worried, and now when I really feel I'm making a decision for myself, you know, something I want to do, something I think will be good for me, fuck it, I get this. Shit.' The word exploded from his mouth. He opened his mouth to say something, but nothing came out. He was shaking his head again. 'I mean, what the fuck am I supposed to do? She was all over the fucking place, she physically held on to me, told me I couldn't go, she needed me. Fuck's sake. She's never needed me, never fucking wanted me. And now. Now when I'm really wanting to do something for me, *for me* . . .' He shook his head again and took a deep breath. 'So now, I don't know, what do I do? I don't know.'

'I'm wondering if you want to stay for her, whether you really think she needs you, where you think she's coming from. And I want to say that I hear how difficult it must have been, not what you expected at all, and I want to acknowledge that it sounds like before all this happened you had kind of a made a decision.'

'I had, but you know, she was being so dramatic. Said she'd kill herself. I don't think she was serious, but she has made attempts back in the past – you know that.'

Helen nodded. Mark's mother was known to the service in the past although before her time there.

'Yeah, so you know she could do it, but, well, I'm going to say something hard here, Mark, but it's because I'm co-ordinating your care, wanting to help you make the choices that are best and right for you. What do you really want? What do you *really* want?'

'I want to get away. No question about that. But I can't. Shit, she's fucked me up before, she's fucking me up again.'

'Sounds pretty clear, you're not going to let her fuck you up again.'

'Yeah, but, what if something happens, what if I go and she does something stupid? I was clear until yesterday.'

'So, the result of yesterday is that you're now feeling you can't go, but you want to go?' Helen was sure she hadn't taken the edge out of her voice – she was feeling pissed off. She could see how important it was for Mark to move, how much he had thought it through but now the histrionics of his mum was threatening to sabotage it.

The discussion continued, and gradually Mark edged more and more back towards his own desire to move on, to make the change. He told her how it felt important for him to spend time around healthy people. He could see how badly he'd been affected by his own family life and how he wanted something different. 'I've been down there, spent time with Rod and it's just so different. So different.' As he continued to speak Mark could feel the anxiety rising within him. Helen noticed how he was looking increasingly tense and she highlighted this. Mark agreed.

She was concerned how he might be left feeling again after the session and asked about what he planned to do next. He said he was unsure, but knew he couldn't go on feeling like this. Said he felt now it was a mistake to have said anything to his mum, wish he'd just got on with it.

By the end of the session Mark was much more in touch with his wanting to move south west, if only for a while to get himself together. He decided that when he felt the time was right, he'd try to convince his mum from the angle that it was temporary, to get his head straight and get his drug use sorted out. But he wanted to get away. But he also again acknowledged that he was finding it helpful getting the support and everything he was getting at the moment and didn't want to end it yet.

Helen suggested that perhaps they should spend time preparing for his moving on, thinking it through a little more? Mark agreed. Said he'd done a lot of that filling in that life line after the last session, but he hadn't brought it with him; in fact he had screwed it up after seeing his mother and it was in the litter bin. He'd dig it out when he got back.

The session was drawing to a close, Helen reminded him of his meeting the next day about the day programme. Mark said he hadn't forgotten, he'd be there. He wanted to try everything to get himself sorted. He left and Helen reflected for a few minutes on her own reactions to Mark's dilemma. She knew she was angry. She realised she didn't really know what was the best move for Mark but it did seem that getting away, if only for a while, made a lot of sense. It was what he wanted to do. He had someone to give him support and a place to live. But what was he going to do with his feelings about his mother? She was shaking her head as she went to the filing cabinet to get out her notes. She was seeing her manager later that day and she wanted to check a few things out with him around the practicalities of transferring a client elsewhere. She wanted to talk it through.

Friday 21 July – day programme preliminary meeting
It was Carrie who Mark saw about the day programme. She seemed pleasant enough, pretty down to earth, seemed sensitive to his apprehension. What she described sounded good. Six weeks, twice a week. Some of it would be therapeutic, looking at why he used, what thinking was associated with it and how he might think differently. There'd be factual sessions on drugs and alcohol, how they affected you. They had a session on overdose risk. Mark mentioned his experience. Carrie hoped he would contribute his experience to the discussion if he felt at ease with that. They'd also be looking at the challenges of change. Mark mentioned that he was considering moving away but wanted to undergo the programme first to get himself ready in himself. Carrie said that it sounded like a positive decision and, yes, that would no doubt come up during the sessions. She also said that they'd look at relapse prevention.

She asked Mark a bit about his own history although she said that they'd got a copy of the initial assessment from Helen. Also asked him what had happened since the assessment to bring her up to date. Also, what his longer-term goals were regarding his drug and alcohol use. Mark explained how he knew he would have to give it up, at least the drugs, probably would want to have the odd drink, but that at the moment all seemed well ahead. At the moment he just wanted to feel stable, keep to his methadone and then, well, at some point think about reducing down. He hoped he'd be able to start that in the not too distant future, but he didn't want to rush anything.

Carrie said she thought that was wise, and she also commented that it was sometimes good to not leave it too long as well. 'People can get into a rut with methadone, find it difficult to contemplate further change. At the moment change is in the air for you, and while I don't think everything should change at once, sometimes you have to keep the momentum? The danger, as you've said, is too much, too soon, and it becomes hard to sustain. So I always think it's a case of slowly, slowly, but maintain an outlook of looking for the next step.'

She described the image of space, said she didn't know if it was technically true but it was an image she often used. 'If a space rocket takes off, if it doesn't keep the power on, well, gravity will pull it back. It has to break away from gravity enough to reach orbit, yeah?'

Mark nodded.

'So you need to break away from the gravitational pull of heroin, and alcohol, and the idea of dealing with things with substances, yeah?'

He could see that.

'And in trying to break free you go through different stages of effort, resolving different things – attitudes, relationships, memories etc. – like stages in a rocket. Each stage moves you a little further away from the lifestyle you've been used to, weakening the thinking and the feelings that will pull you back. But you have to at least get into orbit, but even then, eventually you can still get pulled back in. Hence the analogy goes further; you have to break orbit and go off on your own journey. The rocket goes into outer space; maybe you have to find a different inner space, and, as well, absorb yourself into some new lifestyle, relationships, everything, yeah?'

Mark was nodding. It was a simple image and yet one that Mark could relate to. Yes, he thought, I can see that. 'So going to counselling, the programme here, other stuff, is all helping me on this kind of journey, all stages in that rocket?'

'That's right. And what's important is that we all work together so that we are all working towards sending you in the same direction.'

Mark could see the sense in that. 'So whatever kind of treatment I get is helping me to get where I need to go.'

'That's right.'

'And at the right time for me?'

'Precisely.'

Greater integration between treatment services and modalities is a vitally important feature of Models of Care. Inter- and intra-agency working is crucially important. Everyone engaging with the client on their process of recovery is part of a co-ordinated effort – co-ordinated by the care co-ordinator – to ensure that the client receives what they need and that the integration is maintained as well as relevance to where the client is at. This can mean ensuring that the areas being dealt with at any one time are relevant to the client's needs. For instance, it would not be much good moving a client into a 'Dependency to Work' initiative if they were still chaotic in their drug use and generally unable to get out of bed till after midday. Or imposing a methadone reduction on a client who had barely stabilised and had just witnessed the death of his best friend.

Mark left the session thoughtful. The programme would begin week after next. Carrie said that they were very happy for him to be part of it, that she would call Helen to confirm it that afternoon. Mark explained that she would be re-organising his contact with her to fit around the programme. Said he was looking forward to it, though with some apprehension. 'Haven't done much in groups, I guess.'

'No, apart from family – and it sounds like that wasn't such a good experience. Our other experience of groups is being at school . . .'

'. . . that was a nightmare . . .'

'. . . and being with other people who are using.'

'Yeah, so it's gonna be quite a new experience for me, yeah?'

Carrie nodded and sought to reassure him that while it may seem strange, he'd get used to it and find it helpful.

Mark left, feeling positive. So, next week is the last week with the current set-up, then it changes, and I get ready to go south west. Yes! He knew he had to do it; he knew at some level that what he was doing was right. He also knew it wouldn't be easy; nothing ahead of him was going to be easy. His mind drifted back to that life line he'd drawn with Helen. The fact that the 'carry on using' line was shorter than the 'change your habits' line. OK, no guarantees of anything, but that image had stuck with him – not in the forefront of his mind, but it drifted into focus now and then. Yeah, I want a life, a proper life, make a go of it. He felt positive. The future was uncertain, he knew that but, hell, it couldn't be worse than the past.

Summary

Mark has used again but did not take the methadone. He has explained what happened and still wants to go to his cousin's, which he does, and it is a positive experience for him. The clinic maintains its prescribing regime in spite of Mark struggling to stay with his script. Mark explores his options with Helen through the use of a dividing life line so he can see what positives and negatives there are for change and for not changing. His sensed desire to get away is increasing.

CHAPTER 7

Urging change, preparing for detoxification

- Methadone maintenance (Tier 3)
- Care co-ordination (Tier 3)
- Structured therapeutic counselling (Tier 3)
- Day programme (Tier 2)

Monday 24 July – prescribing clinic

Mark managed to maintain himself on his methadone. They took a urine sample from him to check that there were no other substances being used. Mark had come to accept this now. At first, it had felt like he wasn't trusted but after the occasion a few weeks back when he had used, well, yeah, he understood where they were coming from.

They discussed how his treatment would be re-organised as from the following week. As had been discussed before, Mark would attend the day programme on the Monday, see Helen for a care co-ordination session on the Tuesday, see Tony for therapeutic counselling on the Wednesday, attend the day programme on the Thursday and then see Dr Ashton and Helen on Fridays. They took the opportunity to re-assess the level of methadone and the daily supervised consumption arrangements. Mark said it wasn't always easy, but he didn't want the methadone to start going up. He knew he now had a fuller package of support and treatment and felt he could use this to keep himself stable. The daily supervised consumption made him get up and get out each day, and he'd kind of got used to that now. So that maybe that was a positive result, but he hoped that could change in the future.

Dr Ashton agreed but pointed out that they needed him to be stable over a number of months with no use on top. But they would keep it under review and, obviously, if he was still working towards this when he moved south west, then they would let the other service know so that he didn't have to start the clock again, so to speak.

Mark said that he still did want to go, but he wanted to talk it through further with Helen. Dr Ashton agreed a time to see him a week on Friday in his other clinic, and wished him well with the programme.

They discussed detoxification. Mark wasn't sure. Felt he should stay as he was for a while longer before considering reducing. This was agreed as this would be regularly reviewed. It was all written down and Mark was given a copy.

Care plans need to be constantly reviewed and updated as situations change, and as the client perhaps adjusts their own goals, or in response to crisis. Ensuring that the client has a copy of what has been agreed is also important. It needs to be produced collaboratively so that there is ownership by both the client and the professionals involved.

Care co-ordination session
'As we've reviewed the prescribing maybe we should review everything else, for instance, the counselling. Is it proving helpful?'

Mark nodded. 'Yes, but it's not easy. Doesn't always leave me feeling comfortable, you know, but, yes, it's good to have someone to listen to what you have to say.'

'I know it's confidential, so you don't have to go into more detail than you wish, but I'm wondering what it is that you have been talking about that's been helpful?'

'I feel like I'm sort of just talking about things, my past usually, my drug use, a bit about my hopes for the future, but mainly about the past and stuff. And that's good, yeah, nice to have someone who really kind of, I don't know, takes things on board. I mean, you do too, but, well, he's different. Seems to be happy to let me talk about whatever I want to talk about and yet it always seems what I need to say.'

Helen smiled. That sounded like Tony. She was very aware of the contrasting styles and also the different demands of their roles. As a care co-ordinator, and with a nursing background, she worked to clear protocols in many ways and had a definite agenda with her clients. She had a specific duty to ensure that the client's health needs were being met – physical and mental. Having had both general and mental health experience she knew she was well placed to hold the overview of Mark's health needs. She was very much at ease with her role and felt that she could bring her professional expertise to it to good effect.

Tony, however, could be more freed up in many ways, or at least that was her perspective. She had realised a while back that the role of care co-ordinator couldn't be provided by someone working as a therapist with a client. The power relationship wasn't helpful and she had other responsibilities, things she could be called upon to do on behalf of the client. The therapeutic counsellor did not have any of that. It was a good system, splitting the two functions, hopefully giving the client the best of both worlds.

The care co-ordinator has the overall responsibility of ensuring that the package of care for a given client is designed to meet their needs, is offered and monitored. Drawing on the established protocols and the system of integrated care pathways, she will have established, through collaboration with the client, a range of treatments, support and interventions that will be designed to cater for that particular client. Each package should be unique for each client, based on their needs, their experiences, their current difficulties and their aspirations for the future. Care co-ordination is a demanding role, particularly working with clients who are themselves chaotic or leading risky lifestyles, or simply not engaging consistently with services. Care co-ordinators' caseloads need to be to a level that reflects the complexity of the clients they are working with at any given time.

Yes, she thought, I know my role. Monitor what is being offered, maintain an ongoing assessment of physical and mental health needs, offer motivational interviewing and some applied cognitive-behavioural work to help clients clarify their relationship with their drug use, but the deeper, ingrained relational stuff and the psychological traumatic aspects she left to the therapists to focus on.

'So,' Helen replied, 'the counselling is really helpful. Good. Yes, Tony has a relaxed style and yet he's pretty tuned in as well.'

Mark nodded. 'Yes, I've sensed that. Yes, it's good to unload. And it is helping me make sense of things. I mean, I do think it is helping my motivation. I suppose it's hard to separate out exactly what is making the difference, 'cos everything is really, but he does help me become more aware of feelings, and I'm more aware of how I've been affected by the past, and, yeah, I really want to change. In fact, I know it's more than realise, I know I've got to. I can't remember if it was before or after seeing Carrie at the day programme, but I thought of that life line again – it keeps coming into my mind – and how the "carry on using" line is shorter. You know, it sounds crazy, it's such a little thing, and yet I can't let go of that? It really has got to me. And yeah, I need that, but something so simple.' He shook his head and continued to look Helen in the eyes.

'It is simple, and yet it does make the point, and I guess not having a life that is at risk of being shorter because of the kind of drug use you were involved in, well, it makes the point.' Helen wasn't sure what else to say. Her response sounded a bit convoluted, but she thought she'd said what she wanted, just wished she could have used a few less words.

'So, yeah, that gave me something to think about as well.'

'Anything else about the counselling?'

Mark thought for a moment, folding his hands in his lap and looking up towards the corner of the room, and biting his lip as he did so. His thoughts went back to the last session. 'I was looking out of the window – and, yeah, I've just realised something that is weird. We use the same room, yeah?'

'How do you mean?'

'I see you in the same room as Tony, but with him I always sit in your chair. I mean, I'm aware of it and not sure how it happened that way, but it did, but anyway, yeah, I was sitting there last week and was just, you know, looking out of the window.'

'As one does.' Helen bit her lip, realising that probably wasn't a very helpful response, particularly as Mark seemed to be being serious. She wondered why she'd responded like that, but didn't know, so put it aside.

'Yeah, anyway, and I was kind of watching the world go by and it sort of struck me that there was a world out there that I sort of, well, it's a world I don't belong to, and I need to get involved, get into it, stop being on the . . .' he paused, 'I was going to say on the outside looking in, but I guess I'm also on the inside looking out, inside my drug-using world trying to get into that other world out there.'

'Like you were missing out and want to be part of what you were seeing? Sounds quite profound.'

'It was, it just really struck me how much I needed to move on.' He was looking out of the window again, and in a sense reliving the experience. 'Strange, but yeah, and I don't know whether that was part of the counselling – I mean it was – but it just sort of happened. And that and the life-line thing, yeah, they both really make me aware of what I want.'

'And now it's about making it happen, yeah?'

'Sure is.' He rubbed his eyes, suddenly feeling very tired. 'Sorry. Don't always sleep too good. Bad night last night. Lots on my mind.'

Helen wondered whether to continue with the review or focus on what Mark had just said. She decided to voice her dilemma. 'Just wondering whether you want to talk about what's on your mind, or continue with the review, or,' she had just remembered what they had talked about the previous session, 'look at the advantages and disadvantages of you moving away at some point.'

'That's a lot.' Mark paused. He was aware that there was a lot going on in his head at the moment.

'And there's something else as well, I really need to keep tabs on your alcohol intake too as obviously that needs to be controlled particularly as you are taking the methadone . . .'

'. . . and the overdose risk. Yeah, I know, and respiratory failure. I guess my drinking has slipped up a bit since last week. It's all linked, the idea of moving away, the grief from my mum . . .' He breathed out a long sigh, shaking his head once again. 'A few cans just makes it easier, you know, helps me sleep.'

'Didn't help last night.'

'No, probably hadn't had enough.'

'That kind of alcohol "knock out" sleep isn't really restful, you know. OK, it switches you off, but it isn't quality sleep. And there is the risk, if you were to be sick in the night, a greater risk of choking. '

'Yeah, maybe, but it helps.'

'Your body is used to being sedated, Mark, the heroin and the alcohol, now methadone and the alcohol. You need to slowly acclimatise to less.'

'I need the crap out of my head, Helen; you know when I was with Rod I slept OK. Didn't drink as much, couple of beers, but I kind of felt relaxed down there. Maybe it was the air. I don't know. I felt different. I felt good.'

'Good, it shows that given the right environment and a more relaxed atmosphere you can sleep. What we need to do is help you to manage this while you're here as well. Can you keep track of the alcohol? It's problematic that you are drinking while on the methadone script. We don't want the alcohol getting out of control and becoming a problem in itself,' she paused, remembering the life line, 'and the alcohol on top of the methadone does risk a shorter life line.'

Mark felt like he was being accused of being an alcoholic, which he didn't believe he was. He did drugs. OK, so maybe, yeah, he'd accept that he was a junkie, yeah, but not an alcoholic. No way. But that shorter line also got to him as well.

Helen noticed that Mark didn't look too happy. She guessed it was about the focus on his drinking, but she knew that professionally she needed to know. She also needed to ensure Dr Ashton was aware as he was the prescribing doctor.

'I can see it's uncomfortable, Mark, but a diary of your alcohol intake would be helpful. See if there is anything triggering it that can be resolved.' She reached into her file and took out a weekly drinking diary. 'Have a go with this. One row per day, and a whole lot of columns, time started, time taken up drinking, who with, feelings before, how much consumed, what it cost, feelings after, and general comments. Just to try and help to clarify the pattern.'

'OK.' Mark took it but he wasn't at ease. Still felt that his drinking wasn't such an issue. Yeah, he knew he liked to drink, course he did, didn't most people, but he wasn't an 'alcy', he did drugs 'cos he wanted to, not because he had to.

'You really don't like it, do you?'

'I'm in control of my drinking, you know, I'm not like people you see in the park, cans and bottles all around them.'

'No, but you would have had needles and syringes at one time . . .'

'Fuck it.' Mark's jaw had tightened. He was feeling well pissed off with Helen. What the hell was she about today? She felt like she was on his fucking case.

'Yes, it's hard to accept, but what's the difference? You took your substance out of a syringe; they take it out of a can or a bottle. Trying to feel different. Trying to get away from something. Trying to belong. All kinds of reasons, and it gets out of control. You know that, you don't need to hear me saying it, you know what it's like to have to have a fix, to have to find someone to score.'

Mark had gone quiet. He didn't like what he was hearing. 'Yeah, but, I mean, shit, you think I'm an alcy?'

'No, Mark, no, I don't, but I am concerned that your alcohol use, coupled with your methadone, could cause problems. It enhances the suppressive effect on your body. And we know that the more people drink, the more likely they are to end up dependent on it. We don't want that to happen. We want to help you get stable, that's the point of the methadone, get you stable, get you away from needles and the risk of sharing works, reduce risk of infection, try and keep you physically safe. But we also want to stabilise your mood as well, and alcohol will move that around. Yes, that's going to have its appeal, of course it will. That's how life has been for you for so many years. Rollercoaster. Yes? Know what it's like when you come off a rollercoaster, legs all wobbly, you feel like you're still on it. Might want to get back on to take away the wobble. We want you to get used to being on solid, stable ground, Mark, and you can do it. That shorter life line, you don't want it, you know that. We want, I want, to see you get that new life, and make a real go of it.' As she finished Helen realised she had tears in her eyes.

Mark was stunned, amazed, and deeply touched by the passion that had suddenly emerged from Helen. He wasn't sure what to say. He'd started off feeling bloody irritated, going on again about his drinking. But by the time she'd finished, he was listening. She really seemed to care. Or did she? Nah. Probably saying what she had to say. Probably could turn on the tears for effect; women, cry on you when they want to – that was what he thought anyway. He was far from the truth. Helen did care about her clients, and did care about Mark getting things together. She saw this opportunity for him and she knew, from experience, that often they closed before they were taken advantage of. She knew she had to keep Mark stable and motivated to give him a chance of change.

'Well, I want to make a go of it too. I want to put the gear behind me, you know that, but some days it's bloody hard going. Stuff in my head. Then my mum has a go. Now you have a go.' He went silent.

'I may sound like I'm having a go, Mark, but it's because I know that it is risky drinking on top of methadone, as it is using benzos as well, and I'm not saying you are, but we know that you did in the past. We want to encourage you to stay safe, give yourself a chance of the longer life line, a chance of getting out there, making a go of it.'

Sometimes the client benefits from hearing the professional's genuine concerns for their well-being and desire for them to achieve a more healthy lifestyle. Helen's response has left Mark with much to ponder on. Her reasons for saying what she did should usefully be explored in her own supervision. Professionals from all disciplines are affected by the people they work with, and it can lead to them reacting in surprising ways. Sometimes these will be helpful, sometimes not. Whenever a strong reaction emerges it is important to explore this. It brings up the issue of boundaries between the personal and the professional. Being present as a person in the role of the professional can be valuable. Showing some feeling, some emotion, can strengthen the connection between client and professional. And boundaries need to be watched to ensure that the professional role does not get lost.

Mark was still feeling edgy. Helen was conscious that the session was drawing to a close, and she felt she needed to ensure that the likelihood of Mark going out and drinking on his feelings was minimised. 'Take it easy, Mark, take it easy.' She spoke the words fairly softly, and slowly, trying to reflect the meaning of her request through her tone of voice.

Mark nodded though he remained tight-lipped. He breathed in and held his breath, and as he breathed out said, 'Yeah, OK. I know you're right, but some days, I just find it hard to hold things together. Maybe because the appointment's a little later today and I haven't taken the meth yet. Maybe that's leaving me more sensitive.'

'OK. So, I'll see you Thursday and then the programme Monday. And we'll review things again next Friday.'

'OK, thanks. And I'll see Tony on Wednesday as usual.'

Mark left feeling determined. He had a mixture of feelings and he knew that he had been affected by Helen's passionate words. He knew he'd brushed it aside, but then, well, he wasn't used to hearing anyone being that concerned about his well-being. Apart from Nick and Paula, but they were somehow quieter and laid back. It had made an impact on him; maybe he was worth the effort to change. Maybe he had needed to hear what she had said. He was lost in thought as he headed for the bus stop.

Wednesday 26 July – counselling session

Mark spent time again looking at his past, his drug use, his relationship with his mother, and his hatred for Eric, who'd moved in after his father had left. Mark seemed a little more stressed to Tony, the way he was sitting; he seemed to be holding a lot of tension. He mentioned that he was aware that Mark seemed to be sitting quite stiffly. Mark hadn't really thought about it. It was how he was. Didn't see anything to it. Tony let it go. He had made his observation, and he was aware that he wanted Mark to feel free to be open about whatever he wanted.

It was a few minutes later that Mark mentioned his session with Helen, and how she felt he was struggling with the alcohol and the methadone. How he'd reacted to what Helen had been saying. 'She's sharp, really pushes sometimes, at other times seems far more relaxed about everything. Confuses me. Whereas you're pretty consistent.'

Tony nodded. 'That's how it seems, leaves you confused.' Tony was not going to get drawn into a discussion about a colleague. He would listen, empathise with Mark, seek to be authentically present in the relationship with him and offer him warmth and acceptance, but he wasn't going to get into either a collusion with Mark, or oppose him in his views.

'I mean, I don't know, I come along each time and, well, I talk to her, I talk to you, I talk to her again.'

Tony was nodding and holding a steady eye contact with Mark. 'And . . .?'

'There are days when I just wonder if it's all worth it.'

'And today's one of those days?'

Mark closed his eyes and didn't respond. Some days it just all felt so heavy, so much of an effort. He knew it was probably connected to how much he had drunk the night before, and that certainly felt the case today, but sometimes he just felt so drained of energy. Sometimes he just wished he had a clear head, and then maybe he'd get things together. But he also knew that it would mean him experiencing all kinds of feeling and he really wasn't sure if he could face that.

Tony respected the silence and did not comment further. He waited for Mark.

Working with silence is important. Much can be achieved when seemingly there is little outward communication. However, for the client, a great deal can be going on. By respecting the client's wish for silence by not disturbing it, the client is offered the opportunity to be with what is present within them. And it might be uncomfortable, but that is OK. Sometimes too much

> exchange of words can mean the client avoids what is below the surface. Silence can put them in touch with it, and can move the therapeutic relationship on to a deeper level.

Mark closed his eyes and rested himself back in the chair. His eyes felt heavy. He breathed in slowly. His mind was dulled, no thoughts, just an awareness of his eyes, his breathing and the top of the chair against the back of his head – oh, and his elbows against the arms of the chair. Yes, he did feel stiff. His shoulder blades felt tight; he pulled his shoulders back to try and release the tension, but it didn't make much difference. He sat.

Tony continued to sit and maintain his attention and his attitude of warm acceptance. Mark was no doubt tired, not only physically tired but probably emotionally tired with his struggle to keep to his script. He knew what it could be like. He'd used in the past, long time ago now, but, yes, he knew what it could be like. How difficult it could be. And in his time there weren't the services there were today. He'd sorted it for himself. Realised it wasn't taking him anywhere and had taken control of his life. He wondered about self-disclosing, but it didn't seem relevant. Mark hadn't asked so presumably it wasn't an issue in the forefront of his mind.

> Some people working within drug and alcohol services may have their own experience of drug use (problematic or not). From a personal view, my perception is that this is perhaps more common in services offering Tier 2 interventions. While it can enrich services, it can also present challenges and opportunities. Ex users can bring a wealth of experience and understanding into the role, and often a greater sense of credibility for some clients. Yet, as with all professionals working in the area of substance misuse, their own personal attitudes towards drug users and drug use need to be clear. The establishing of national standards for training in working with this client group is important to ensure that problems of attitude are resolved. For Tony, his knowledge stemming from his own drug use can help him more fully appreciate Mark's struggle, yet at the same time it could leave the clarity and accuracy of his empathy affected by his own experiences and make it difficult for him to let Mark know that he has heard his particular experience.

Mark yawned, opened his eyes and blinked. 'Did I doze off?'

'I don't think so, but you looked as though you had relaxed into the chair.'

'Hmm, still feeling tight, you know.' He stretched his shoulders again but the tightness remained.

'Tight?'

Mark nodded.

'Pain, isn't it?'

'Sure is.' He paused. 'Helen would blame the alcohol.'

'Mhmm, that's what you feel she'd say if she was here.'

'It isn't just that. I really don't want to get a problem with alcohol. I see people like that, I'm not like that. Helen thinks I am.'

Tony felt a surge of surprise. Mark hadn't really given the impression to him of having a huge alcohol problem. 'You say that Helen thinks you have a big alcohol problem?'

'Yeah.'

'And I take it you don't think you have?'

'No. Just like a few cans, you know?'

Tony knew, and he knew about the dangers of drinking while on methadone. He was sure Helen and Dr Ashton would have pointed that out. His dilemma now was whether he added his voice to this, and therefore appeared to side with the others in a way that Mark might interpret as being against him, or did he say nothing and run the risk of appearing to contradict what might be being said. He decided to maintain his empathy and not get caught up in taking sides, though he could sense the temptation. He knew he needed to be particularly self-aware and that it was maybe an issue for his own supervision.

'Mhmm, just a few cans. Doesn't feel like a problem to you?'

'Helen says it is.'

'And you don't agree?'

Mark shrugged.

Tony said nothing, simply allowed Mark to be with his thoughts and feelings. He didn't feel any need to press him on the point; rather he wanted to offer acceptance towards Mark, not necessarily to agree with him, but to accept his right to his own view.

Mark was feeling tense, wound up, though he didn't have anything he could put it down to. Hadn't really settled after his mother's reaction to his idea of moving away. That still wound him up.

'Just don't like people on my case.'

'People, what, telling you what to do, what's best for you in their view?'

'Yeah, that kind of stuff. I've not got a drink problem, just like a few cans, you know?'

'Yes, I hear you, Mark, it's not a problem to you how much you drink.'

'And Helen thinks it is.' He felt like saying, 'bitch', but didn't.

'Mark, I really do sense that you don't like hearing what Helen is saying, and I guess I'm wanting to clarify something here for my own understanding. Is she concerned about how much you are drinking, or the simple fact that you are drinking given that you are on the methadone?'

'I know about that. People do drink with it, you know?'

'I know, lots of people do, and it does increase risk.'

Tony has effectively stepped out of his counselling role and it could be heard by Mark that he is taking sides. In fact, Tony didn't need to say anything other than a minimal response and a short empathic reflection: 'Mhmm, people do drink with it.'

Mark scratched his head with his left hand – with attitude. He was feeling angry, pissed off, just felt like he'd had enough. 'I'm pissed off, fucking pissed off.'

Tony could see and hear the anger in Mark's tone of voice. It felt very present. He raised his own voice a little to match him. 'So you're pissed off about it all, yeah, fucking angry.'

'Bloody well am.' He lapsed back into silence, and started picking at the arms of the chairs with what little he had left of his well-chewed finger nails. 'Just want to get away from it all, from every-fucking-thing. Oh God . . .' He turned to look out of the window. He could see cars driving past, their occupants seemingly living to some purpose. He had no purpose, drifting, what he'd done all his life, or so it seemed. Drifting from one hit to the next. He wasn't in the place he had been looking out of the window in that earlier session. He was just fed up, feeling shut out.

'Tough time, tough feelings, huh?'

Mark took a deep breath and blew the air forcefully back out through his nose. 'Fucking tough time.' He could feel the tension in his arms and shoulders, and it felt as though a headache was coming on as well. He blew out another deep breath and slumped back in the chair. 'Shit.' He closed his eyes. Tony remained attentive but said nothing to disturb Mark's internal process. 'I'm tired of it all, Tony, I really am.' He opened his eyes. 'I want a life, God knows I want a life. I feel so fucked up with it all. And I don't think the methadone helps. I mean, I feel like it's clouding me all the time. Yeah, helps to stop me feeling things, but they come back. I can't use more, I've got to learn to handle them. I guess that's what the day programme will be all about.' He yawned. 'I am just so tired of it all.' He was still slumped back in the chair; now he was shaking his head. He had closed his eyes again.

'That tiredness is really overwhelming. Tired of it all, tired of the methadone, tired of how things are.' Tony had noticed how the anger had diminished. The atmosphere felt flatter suddenly, heavy, like everything was an effort. He felt it in himself as well.

The session continued slowly. Mark's tiredness really slowed him down. He thought it might be the methadone kicking in – he'd taken his daily dose earlier, but it didn't feel like it was that. He knew that kind of lethargy; this was different. It felt total. He could hardly lift his head off the chair back. 'I need to head off to sleep, Tony, I really do.'

Tony nodded in agreement. 'Yes, seems like you need a rest, and I am also mindful that sometimes tiredness can be linked to a psychological process as well. You've got so much you're tired of, and so much you want to change in your life.'

'Yeah, if I can. I sometimes wonder *what is the point?*'

'Mhmm, what is the point?' Tony kept his empathic response accurately reflective of what Mark had said, using the same tone of voice as well.

'Because I want more than the crap I've had.'

'Mhmm, want something a lot better?'

'Yeah, better than what I've had to live through. As far back as I can remember . . .' He took a deep breath and again breathed the air out forcefully. He sat forward in the chair; he was stiff but his head felt a little clearer, and he felt the anger had lessened. 'What's the point? Doesn't matter how much I talk about it, I've got to do something. I will move on, Tony, I will get through this, I'm bloody determined to.'

Tony empathised with his tone of voice. 'Bloody determined to.'

Yeah, Mark thought, I am, I just lose it sometimes, drift again, feel frustrated, but I can't stay like that. 'I want things to be better. I want a clearer head. I'm going to talk to Helen about switching to something else. I gather there's something else available, buper . . . something, can't remember what it's called.'

'Buprenorphine?'

'Yeah, that sounds like it. I was against the idea before but I just wonder if the methadone is leaving me too foggy sometimes. I'm seeing her tomorrow. You don't know anything about it?'

'Only a little I've read. There are some information booklets around, but talk to Helen, she can give you the information you need. It sounds like a positive move, wanting a clearer head.'

'I have to, Tony, I've got to get a grip of things and I can't do that like this. I need to get myself together.'

The session moved on to Mark exploring his need to get himself together, and though he couldn't clearly imagine what it would be like, he knew it had to be better, and he knew it was the only way forward. The tiredness had passed and they discussed this as well; it was as though his affirmation of needing to move on, of getting himself together, somehow helped to lift it.

The session drew to a close. Mark remained motivated to discuss changing his medication and, perhaps more importantly, in touch with his experienced need to get his head clear. Tony felt good about the session. A lot of feelings, it was good that they were being expressed and allowed to be without judgement. He wondered how feelings would have been handled in Mark's early years. He guessed it was probably the case that they were expressed forcefully, and probably quite loudly, leaving Mark perhaps with a tendency to normalise loud and uncontained expression of feelings and also anxiety about losing it when feelings were running high.

He sat back in the chair and took a deep breath himself. Tiring session, he thought. He realised how much he had been concentrating and took himself off for a walk in the fresh air, taking a cup of water with him as he went past the water dispenser.

Thursday 27 July – care co-ordination

Helen reviewed Mark's progress. He was more motivated and he was wondering about getting off the methadone and on to buprenorphine, or Subutex as it is branded. He'd heard about it, but it seemed some people found it good, others found it really hard to get on to. 'Lot of people trading it, making up their own cocktails.'

'Yeah, we know, and we're trying to contain that.'

'Do you think that would be the best way to get off the methadone?'

They discussed the options. Mark didn't feel stable enough to seriously reduce his current prescription. So it would have to be a case of transferring across. Mark said he'd heard some people seemed to switch to heroin and then reduce, that for some it was an easier transition.

Helen said that wasn't an option – they weren't prescribing heroin and they weren't going to encourage him to use off the street. She thought it was probably as much to do with people having negative feelings about methadone anyway. 'It's really a matter of support. What we've learned is that we need to give people the same amount of support when they are transiting across as we would for someone who is detoxing. So, we'd be seeing you daily and you could call in during those first few days. The thing is, at the moment, it could disrupt your day programme.'

'Hmm, like I might not be OK to go?'

'Yes, and they might not want you to be in the group if you're getting a bad reaction.'

They discussed it further and Mark said he'd check it out the next day when he went to the day programme. He said he wanted to give it a go. He knew it wouldn't be easy, that, yeah, he'd be more aware of feelings and stuff, but he knew he had to be. Felt he wanted to get himself clearer before he went south west.

Helen agreed to have a chat with Dr Ashton when he was in on Friday as well, and then they could all talk about it when she saw him the next Tuesday.

Friday 28 July – prescribing clinic
'Mark's interested in buprenorphine; what do you think?'

Dr Ashton nodded. 'To get off the methadone, presumably, but does he want maintenance or to detox?'

'We didn't really discuss that. I said I'd talk to you about it and then discuss his options with him next week.'

'Well, I wouldn't prescribe for maintenance. We start doing that, then more will get out on the street, and, well, we'll end up with the problems we have with methadone being so available being transferred to buprenorphine. I chatted to Phil recently, said that it was getting used a lot on the street; some people are using it to detox themselves but there are a few crushing it up and injecting, unfortunately.' Dr Ashton shook his head. Over the years he'd seen the horrible effects of injecting crushed tablets. That was the last thing he wanted to see more of. 'I'd be happy to prescribe for a detox for Mark, but I think maybe you need to spend time talking that through with him.'

Helen nodded. 'He's also unsure what they'd feel about this on the day programme. He's asking them today.'

'Shouldn't be a problem. Some people react; they can get a precipitated withdrawal reaction if they take too much the first day. What's Mark on at the moment?'

'35 ml.'

'So, maybe OK, just about. Wouldn't do it above 40 ml, prefer closer to 30. At least he has lots of support and if they're OK at the day programme that will help. We could start him on a Monday – get him to pick up before the day programme starts and then, what, you see him on Tuesdays, or will do now?'

Helen nodded.

'So it could work out. Have a chat with him Tuesday. It would mean slowly detoxing him over three to four weeks, but he's motivated, and he's certainly getting the support at the moment, and maybe the timing with the day programme would work really well. It just depends how they feel about him detoxing on the programme. But if he takes it slowly, well, I think he should be OK. And we can keep him on daily pick-up, but he'll need to appreciate that he should only take what he feels he needs. Not everyone needs the 12 mg I'd normally prescribe, so, probably give him 12 mg but get him to take 4 mg and see how he goes, and take another 4 mg if he starts feeling withdrawals coming on, and he's got the other 4 mg just in case. Psychologically, knowing it's there can reduce some of the anxiety. Quite a few can hold at 8 mg, and then we can start the reduction.'

'I'll also get out an information leaflet for him as well.'

'OK, so we'll discuss it again when I see him next Friday.'

Monday 31 July – day programme 1
Mark attended the day programme. He'd stopped off at the clinic on the way for his daily methadone, and he was glad for that. Though he was trying to be quite confident, underneath he was anxious about it, unsure quite what he was letting himself in for. He knew that it was good for him – at least, that was what he kept telling himself. The day began with a round of introductions, to get people talking. He was paired up with Judy, and they had to spend a few minutes each talking about themselves, why they were on the programme. Judy was a cocaine user, very different world from that of Mark. She'd had a well-paid job in the city, but there had been financial problems where she worked. She hadn't been able to maintain her expensive habit after she had lost her job. She was still using a little, 'recreationally, of course', and she added, 'I can take it or leave it', though the truth was she had generally took it and rarely left it.

She'd got a boyfriend and they had been living together, but she had moved out for a while 'to get her head straight' and was living with her sister. Her boyfriend used heavily and wasn't keen to do anything about it. Judy, though, had been persuaded to come on the programme. Since moving out she had been changing, and her life was settling down. She couldn't afford to use, and her sister kept an eye on her. She'd always got on well with her sister, and she never used anything. Just liked to go out and about and enjoy herself without using substances. Judy was beginning to adjust.

Mark told her about himself, saying that he was trying to restart his life, get some control back. Said he found time hung heavily for him and he'd been encouraged to take the programme as part of his weekly structure of support. Said he was pleased to be there and tried to hide his anxiety.

They were then moved into groups of four and each introduced the other to the two new participants. As this process unfolded Mark began to feel a little more relaxed. A couple of the people he'd seen at the clinic – they were also getting daily methadone. And someone else he'd seen some other time, he wasn't sure when.

The rest of the morning was taken up with discussion around what people's expectations were, what they hoped for from the course and what they were anxious about. It seemed like there were a lot of different views. Mark had sort of assumed everyone was there to 'get a life', which is one of the things he'd said. Some sounded like they were where he was; others just wanted a break from whatever they were using and had been encouraged to come along to help them get to the point of deciding to reduce their use or stop. There was also some ambivalence around as well. Seemed like a couple were there because they'd convinced their drug workers that they wanted to change, but already they didn't seem too bothered. Quite a mixed bag, Mark thought to himself. He felt pissed off that some might only be there for the ride, but he said nothing.

Brian gave an overview of the programme, how it was structured, what was expected of the participants. Carrie then talked about confidentiality and they devised a set of 'ground rules'. Mark smiled to himself thinking, yeah, this bunch of fuckers won't respect that. He didn't voice his thoughts, but made a mental note to be a little wary of what he said about himself. The drug-using community is a small world. He'd want to feel really sure he could trust the others, and he doubted that he ever would. One of the topics highlighted was relationships with other members of the programme. The facilitators advised that sexual relations were better avoided, that people trying to maintain control or reduce could be vulnerable, and the programme wasn't there to sort out relationship problems that developed outside of the group. They had enough to focus on without that affecting the group process. Seemed fair enough to Mark. Yeah, he had realised he fancied a couple of the other participants, but he wasn't planning to get involved.

The rest of the day involved an information session – Carrie and Brian, the facilitators, both talking about different drugs. There was a questionnaire about the effects of drugs and how risky they might be, and how addictive they were. They also listed all the different drugs that participants were using and had used in the past. Seemed pretty comprehensive – certainly didn't look like anything was missing. Quite a mix of stimulant users and depressant users, with a few favouring the more trippy experiences. And Mandy, who looked a real mess, seemed to have used everything. She sort of seemed to drift in and out in herself. Shit, what a state, Mark thought. And yet there was something about her that made him smile. She'd survived it all – so far, anyway.

Some of the participants were working, though none were full-time. Generally bits of work when they could get it. Everyone else was either registered unemployed or on the sick, except for Lucy – who preferred to be called Lu – whose partner worked and she was simply at home during the day and used dope to blank out her past.

At the end of the day, Mark felt a bit more relaxed. It had felt good, but he did feel tired. Sitting around obviously had that effect. A lot had gone on, a lot to focus on, a lot to think about. He headed off, taking the same bus as Mandy. She told him she was going to use, did he want to come along, share the experience. Mark was tempted, bit of female company, but he knew that wasn't going to help him. A few months back, he'd have been up for it, been up for anything. But now? No. He was in another place. Yeah, it was tempting, but no. Told her he had to get back to meet up with friends. She got off before his stop. She seemed a little pissed off with him but, well, he felt sorry for her. The thought crossed his mind, 'maybe I could help her'. He'd like to do that; the thought felt good. Maybe he'd spend time with her next week.

Tuesday 1 August – care co-ordination
'Yeah, I'm enjoying it. Seems an interesting bunch of people.' Mark described to Helen his experience of the day programme, and how it was going. 'I mean, only first session and, yes, I was anxious, but I soon found my place.' He said a little more about the different people on it. He also talked about Mandy, and what had happened on the way home.

Helen was experiencing alarm bells in her head. She had learned to trust them, although the facts spoke for themselves. Mark, trying to stay clean, and Mandy, openly planning to use.

'Do you think it will help you in achieving your goals to spend time with Mandy?' She didn't want to tell him what was good for him, not at first, anyway. She wanted to encourage him to think it through, weigh up the pros and cons for himself.

'How do you mean?'

'Sounds like she's still using. How do you feel about that?'

'I wish she wasn't. Maybe I can help her?'

'Maybe.' Helen left her comment in the air for Mark to mull over.

Mark was feeling irritated. 'So, you think I shouldn't spend time with her then?'

'Well, to be absolutely honest, no, I don't, not at this stage in your own process of trying to keep in control of your drug use, Mark. And, yeah, I appreciate that that's not easy to hear, but I want to be honest with you.'

Coming off substances is a vulnerable time. Feelings can run high, feelings that may be new to the person, and which can be overwhelming. Also, there is the risk of becoming dependent on a person, using the relationship to escape from other areas of one's life and the feelings associated with them. The problematic risk is heightened when the other person is using in a more problematic way, the risk being that, in this case, Mark is drawn back into a pattern of use that he is seeking to move away from.

'Hmm.' Mark did not feel very comfortable and he felt angry. He knew Helen was concerned for his best interests; she'd made that clear in earlier sessions.

'Mark, I don't want to tell you what to do, and you must make your own decisions, but I simply want to express my concern. Do you need that kind of temptation at this time? I don't want you to slip up, Mark. I'm not saying you will, you probably won't, but it's about risk factors, and for you to be with people that are using at the moment ups the risk.'

Mark could see that. And he also felt he wanted to help Mandy. She seemed so vulnerable, somehow. He wanted to help. But he was uneasy about it now. Yeah, he didn't want to mess up, but he didn't want to be told what to do in his private life either.

'OK, maybe you're right.' Mark wasn't convinced but he wanted to get off the subject.

For Helen, Mark had capitulated too easily. Her experience in working with people told her that sometimes people just wanted to get the professional off their case and would say anything.

'Mandy'll get support from the facilitators and from her own care co-ordinator and whatever treatment that has been planned for her. She's probably at a different stage of change to you. I want to see you get this programme done, get yourself detoxed via the Subutex script and on your way to a new life.' Helen sought to bring Mark back to his focus, his goals, and maybe then he'd gain a fresh perspective on things. She wanted to ensure that he gave himself the best chance of maximising the benefits and the potential from the planned care that was available to him. 'You're on the programme for you, Mark. Bottom line.'

'Yeah, I am there for me.' Mark felt himself relax a little. He was thinking, maybe she's right. Maybe it'll just complicate things. But he felt for Mandy as well.

They continued to discuss the situation, and Mark realised increasingly that his own recovery was his priority. Yeah, he could see that.

They moved on to the matter of the Subutex. Helen conveyed her conversation with Dr Ashton. They also agreed that she would speak to one of the day programme facilitators, to check out their view of having someone on the programme who was detoxifying.

Helen brought up the topic of the drinking. Mark hadn't brought his diary, but he did say that he'd had a couple of evenings when he'd had four cans of 5% lager, otherwise he'd drank less, and not every night. He hadn't drunk after the group, but he had done after their last care co-ordination session, and he explained it was because he'd felt irritated by it all. In fact, the heavier nights had been at the end of the last week; he'd been better with it since then. They explored this. It was clear that part of Mark's alcohol use was around simply feeling uncomfortable about things, about anything. He realised, perhaps a little more clearly, just how he was used to using alcohol to get away from feelings, as he had with heroin before.

They went back to Subutex and Helen raised the issue of what effect it would have on Mark if he lost some of the haziness that the methadone had been giving him, and his feelings became more present?

Mark had to accept she had a point, but he knew that he had to take that risk, somehow. And he was able to accept that she was right to be concerned. 'I've got to use the support, the programme, to work it through. I know it won't be easy, but it's what I have to do. It's the days when something gets to me, those are the ones I have to watch.'

Helen mentioned a list of helplines and she gave him the details should he want to use them if, say, he was having a bad evening. He took the list. He could see the sense in that.

Wednesday 2 August – counselling
The counselling session didn't flow too well for Mark. He kind of didn't know what to talk about for the first part of the session. Said he'd talked to Helen, and sorted a few things out. He talked about the day programme again. As he spoke he began to

realise that he wanted to talk about Mandy again. It hadn't gone away. He could still feel he wanted to help her in some way. He knew what conclusion he'd come to with Helen, but he kind of wanted a second opinion.

Mark talked about it, and tried to encourage Tony to agree that there would be no harm in it. Tony maintained his empathy for Mark, simply letting him know what he was hearing, the nature of the dilemma and how Mark seemed to want someone to tell him that it was OK for him to spend time with Mandy.

'So you think it's OK, then?'

Human nature: one person indicates to us that what we are contemplating doing isn't a good idea, but because we feel an urge to continue we seek some-one else to give us the OK. The fact that Mark is now raising this with Tony is a good sign. Mark is unsure, otherwise he would just do it and tell no-one.

Tony could feel a resistance in himself and he recognised that this was a reflex to experiencing being pushed. He didn't have any intention of giving Mark permission to do anything. His role was to hear what Mark was saying and help him make sense of himself, not to advise him what to do.

'You really want to push me to give you my blessing?'

Mark scowled back. 'You're not going to, are you?'

'I'm not here to give you advice or tell you what to do. Sure, talk it through with me, and maybe we can come to greater clarity as to what it is all about. I'm here to listen and enable you to explore yourself, make sense of who you are, your choices.'

Mark sighed.

'It's a tough one for you, isn't it? And part of you is asking about it rather than you just saying nothing and acting on instinct, as it were.' Tony sought to empathise with what he sensed to be Mark's struggle. The sigh had seemed heart-felt. He wanted to let Mark know that he appreciated the potency of what was going on for him. And he wanted to acknowledge that Mark was choosing to raise the issue.

'Yeah. I just want to help, you know?'

'Yeah, I know. Help, make something or someone better, yeah?'

Mark nodded.

Tony maintained silence and kept his attention on Mark, and held in his own heart and mind the intensity of the struggle that he sensed to be taking place within Mark. He could see clearly how it seemed that Mark's head was saying one thing, his heart another. He decided to voice what was present for him, or at least offer it as his sense of what was happening for Mark.

'Seems like your head is saying one thing, and your heart is being pulled in another direction.'

Mark took a deep breath. 'Yeah.' He paused. 'Somehow, she seems very alone, and struggling, and, well, I know what that's like.'

Tony nodded. 'Yeah. And it's horrible, yeah?'

Mark took another deep breath and let it out with a sigh. 'Yeah.'

'Hmm. Yeah.' He said nothing more, but waited, holding within himself a feeling of warmth towards Mark, and an openness to accepting whatever Mark decided to do. Yeah, he could imagine what logically seemed right for Mark, and there was also a vulnerable, needy part of Mark that could be touched by someone like Mandy. He remembered a phrase he'd read recently, 'joined at the wound'. Summed it up, at least, something like that, the sense that people's similar hurt could kind of resonate between them and draw them together. Mark was feeling a huge pull towards Mandy. But was it her, or his own woundedness that was drawing him?

This 'joined at the wound' idea is an important one to bear in mind when working with people with dependencies where relationship issues are involved. People with similar hurts can be drawn together. There is a sense of mutual understanding. It can be helpful, but it can be that it simply means that mutual woundedness is the main attraction and therefore this has to be maintained to keep the relationship alive.

Mark was replaying images from his own past. His own struggle, his own sense of confusion, of doing what he had to in order to get by. He didn't know all of Mandy's background but he kind of guessed it would be similar to his own, maybe worse. He swallowed and took another deep breath. He was feeling really hot.

Tony conveyed his empathy by also taking a deep breath while tightening his lips as he kept his eyes on Mark who had looked up and caught his eye although he hadn't said anything.

Mark was feeling . . . he didn't know what he was feeling, but wasn't comfortable. 'Ohh, shit.'

'Mhmm?'

'I feel like my guts are spinning and yet I feel kind of nothing as well. Like there's so much inside churning around and yet outside I'm kind of numb. I feel kind of buzzy.'

Tony nodded. Yes, he thought, you're probably touching into some deep stuff here. Tony had noticed his own concentration increase. He was aware of feeling much more alert; it seemed to be a really important moment. He didn't say much in response, didn't want to take Mark away from his own inner experience. He moved his hand to his own stomach. 'Spinning,' he paused, and then continued, 'and numb, and buzzy.'

Mark was beginning to feel very light-headed; in fact, he wondered if he was going to faint. He took another deep breath and blew the air out of his mouth. He knew he didn't want to stay with what he was experiencing. And yet it seemed to hold him, like he was psychologically unable to move.

Tony did not want to disturb him. He trusted Mark's process, that his own being knew what was needed and he didn't need to rationalise it. He accepted it and stayed with it, maintaining his openness to his own experience and his warmth and sensitivity towards Mark.

Mark blinked and moved his head slowly. He was aware of feeling stiff. His shoulders seemed locked. He moved them to free them off. It felt a little better, and he felt himself moving away from what had been happening for him.

'What was that about?'

'Seems like you touched into an area of yourself that in its own way was quite powerful.'

Mark shook his head, and drew a deep breath. 'Never felt anything like that before.'

'A new experience, yeah?'

Mark nodded. 'Yeah. Ooh.' He swallowed. 'And yet I feel calmer somehow.'

'Mhmm, that happens, like a storm blows and then it calms again.'

'Yeah.' He paused, reflecting on it. 'Yeah.'

The session drew gently to a close. Mark asked Tony again about Mandy.

'Mark, all I can say is think about what you just experienced. You've got some deep experiencing within you, and it seems that there is something about Mandy that triggers it off, yeah?'

'Yeah, and I can't go there, not yet, not out there. I wouldn't feel safe.'

'Mhmm. So here is a safe place, yeah, but out there, and with Mandy, maybe not so safe.'

'No, not so safe.' He paused before continuing. 'This is heavy stuff. Heavy stuff. And I guess I have to go through it, don't I?'

'Well, it's what is coming up for you at the moment, Mark.'

'Yeah, I need to watch myself.'

Mark left in a very thoughtful mood, very concentrated and yet in a way that seemed unfamiliar to him.

During the afternoon Helen phoned the day programme and spoke to Brian. 'So, how do you feel about Mark being switched to Subutex while on the programme?'

'We're OK with it so long as he has enough support, and it's timed to minimise the impact on the group process.'

'We'd start him on a Tuesday morning, keep an eye on him here, and try and make sure he only takes what he needs. Hopefully he'll be feeling stable for the Thursday.'

'And is it a reduction you're then planning?'

'We need to talk that through but, yes, we don't want to get people being maintained on Subutex and turn it into another methadone. We want to keep it for detoxification, not start sending out the wrong message.'

'Fair enough. We've heard it's on the streets anyway, and, yes, some of the hardened users are messing around with it, even crushing it up to inject, so, yes, we don't want more of it out there than necessary.'

'No. So we'll be talking about it with Mark on Friday and if it seems OK then maybe we'll start it Tuesday although I'd prefer to talk it through with him and plan it but we also want to maximise the opportunity he has with the support he's getting at the moment.'

'Sometimes we just have to go with it and so long as he is supported and encouraged, and isn't under- or over-prescribed, maybe the time is right.'

The conversation continued and it was agreed that any concerns that arose would be discussed again. Helen was keen to ensure that while they were from two separate teams, and one was statutory, the other non-statutory, they maintain good communication. She saw this as a key feature of her role.

Thursday 3 August – day programme 2
The day programme went well, though one of the guys didn't turn up. The facilitators didn't know why. They let his care co-ordinator know, who said that he would call him and check it out, and encourage him to come next time if he was unsure about continuing. Another arrived late – he'd overslept. He was on a methadone script but had used gear since the last session and had drunk heavily, and was out of it. Mark was struck by the fact that the facilitators didn't give him hell. He'd have expected that if he'd done that. But they listened to what he had to say, seemed genuinely concerned that he was OK, checked that he felt well enough to be there and asked if they could use his experience as a learning theme. He agreed.

The morning was then spent on looking at overdose risks – Mark realised he knew some of it, from what he remembered when he was in hospital. He mentioned this and ended up talking about his experience of overdosing. He felt quite good that he seemed to know more than anyone else. He was actually surprised how much he had retained as well.

Throughout the morning he was aware of having to fight the urge to glance over to Mandy. He was very aware of her presence in the group, but he also knew he wanted to keep his focus on the topic. He knew after that last counselling session that he had to look after himself, that there were parts of himself that could get out of control. He knew he hadn't felt he had much control in that counselling session.

In the afternoon they focused on the thoughts and feelings that led up to a using decision. After a talk by Carrie and some examples of how you could turn an experience into an opportunity to use, they broke up into pairs and worked on breaking down their decision-making process. Mark recognised that for him his decision to use was often linked to not feeling in control, of feeling backed into a corner over something, feeling powerless. He'd use to get away from it all. It was an interesting contrast to the guy he was working with, who wasn't an opiate user, but went for speed and cocaine, wanting to feel good, strong, invincible, he called it. Totally different reaction and yet they found their motives were similar. Mark found it fascinating. Wondered why he hadn't done that.

During the discussion period after they'd fed back what had been discussed, he mentioned it. There followed a discussion in which people contrasted their backgrounds and their drugs of choice. Some people simply used anything and everything; at least they had in the past though they were trying to be more in control now, hence being on the programme. Mandy was one of them. Mark had been more of an opiate user. They didn't come up with any great insight on it all, seemed to be so many factors, and also what the dealer had available. Some people had progressed through substances; others had stayed with one drug. But everyone was concerned with moving their mood around, changing how they felt, how they experienced themselves, life, the universe – well, anything and everything. Boredom, frustration, get away from bad memories, get away from what was happening at the time, or the anticipation of what was to come. Yeah, and it felt good. Everyone agreed, yeah, they enjoyed their drugs.

The session ended with a sharing of what people had gained from the day. Mark went back to the start of the day. He hadn't really let go of his reaction to the guy who was out of it. He'd only got told off, and he realised that was what he had expected. But they hadn't. They'd helped him explain what had happened, and he'd agreed to stay around and take it easy. They'd contacted his care co-ordinator who said she was seeing him the next day and would offer support and encourage-ment, and try and help him to keep himself more together for the next session.

No-one in the group wanted him to have to leave. They all felt, yeah, that could be me next time. I wouldn't want to be thrown out. I'd want to be listened to. For a moment the thought had passed through Mark's head – almost worth getting stoned to get a bit of TLC! He knew it wasn't the way, but the thought had crossed his mind.

Mark didn't catch the same bus as Mandy. He left, walking the other way and went into the park. Wanted time to think, to reflect on it all.

Friday 4 August – prescribing clinic and care co-ordination
Mark described his week, the group, how he'd had a heavy counselling session. They discussed the idea of switching him to the Subutex. Mark said he was keen to do it, and he was aware that he had a lot going on for him at the moment. The day programme was giving him a lot to think about, and so was the counselling. And part of him wanted to feel maybe a little clearer in himself, and another part wanted to feel the methadone maybe taking the edge off things.

'So, you're not sure, Mark?' Dr Ashton felt he wanted Mark to feel secure in his decision, whichever way it went. He knew in himself that he didn't know what was for the best. He was inclined though, where there was hesitation, to believe that the time might not be right.

'I want to do it, it's just, well, I've heard some people find it a difficult switch over.'

It was Helen who responded. 'Some do say that, and we'd make sure we had a lot of contact with you, Mark. I mean, for instance, if you started it on a Tuesday morning, you could be here that day, and the next. Bring some magazines in, we can put videos on in one of the rooms for you. Bring something along yourself to watch.'

Services need a range of accommodation and diversions for people who are going to spend all day in the clinic. They need their own space. The environ-ment can be quite intense at times and for a person undergoing a change of medication or a detoxification there is a need for calmness. Sensitivities can be heightened leaving the person more reactive to their surroundings or thoughts that enter their heads. So a place where they can relax, have things to focus their attention on, and for staff to keep an eye on them and monitor them is vitally important.

'How long would it be for, the time on the detox?'

Dr Ashton responded, 'About four weeks to get you down and off, Mark.'

Mark nodded. 'So, I'd just have one more week of the programme left. And then, get away. Yeah, yeah, that could work out.' He looked across to Helen, and then back to Dr Ashton. 'I've got to go for it. It feels like a real opportunity. Then when I get away it'll be drug-free. New start.' He stopped and felt anxious. 'I will get support the other end, won't I?'

Helen nodded. 'I'll talk to them and put through a formal referral. They'll probably want you to talk to them as well. Maybe we can do that on Tuesday, call them while you're here for your session.'

Mark nodded. 'Yeah, just want to be sure, you know?'

'Yeah, that's OK. We'll sort that out.'

Dr Ashton explained about Subutex, what the regime would be. How he'd need to spend time at the clinic on Tuesday so they could monitor and encourage and support him.

'You can bring a video in if you want to watch it; we can set up one of the rooms here. I don't think we are starting anyone else off next week on it, but there are people around. If you can come in first thing Tuesday morning we'll start you off and see how you do during the day. We can let you have more if you feel you need it, up to a maximum of 12 mg. You'll be OK. It's pretty straightforward.' Dr Ashton was keen to reassure Mark. He knew from experience that client expectation could contribute to either a bad or a good experience in these circumstances. He wanted Mark to feel at ease with the process when he came in on Tuesday. He only wanted Mark to have enough to take out any withdrawal reaction from the methadone, hold him stable for a few days – probably until the next week, and then reduce him down slowly. Some of it would depend on how much Mark found he needed to feel stable. They would have to build his dose up until he was stable. He also explained that he needed Mark to be clear of methadone use, that he should take his last methadone early on the day before they began the Subutex prescribing. They would then begin the Subutex when he was beginning to experience withdrawal; otherwise it could cause a precipitated withdrawal reaction.

They moved on to check with Mark that what he was receiving in terms of his treatment and support was OK and helpful. Mark confirmed that it was, but that the counselling was heavy going this past week. Said he definitely knew he needed to continue it when he moved. Helen confirmed she would mention that, and try to make sure it was someone with the same approach. She wanted to be reassured that Mark felt up to the medication switch and the reduction given the 'heavy going' that he had referred to. Did he want to ease off the therapeutic counselling and start again after the move? Mark confirmed that he wanted to stick with it. He liked Tony, liked how he was and though it was hard he somehow knew it was important. Tony seemed to help him explore himself and, yeah, it was uncomfortable at times, but he felt it was important. Helen accepted what he had to say, but also requested that he let her know if, for any reason, it felt like it was too much given that the switch in medication may leave him more sensitive to feelings, and certainly he would feel that way as he reduced.

'I think it's time to start to get to know myself, Helen. I've been clouded in drugs for too long. This isn't just about getting control over drug use, not any more, it's about getting a life. I know it's not going to be easy. I'd like a quick fix – always have! That's been my problem! No, I need to have time with people, healthy people, who can help me find the right direction – you, Tony, Dr Ashton, Carrie, Brian – you're all playing a part in this.'

Helen acknowledged what Mark was saying and the session drew to a close with Helen confirming that she would speak to the other service early next week and get him referred. She'd feed back to him at their next session.

Summary

Helen encourages Mark to think about his alcohol use, and expresses her concern and her wanting him to give himself a chance for change. He finds it hard to hear that his alcohol use is problematic. He attends the counselling and realises how tired he is of it all, how much he wants to change. He mentions Subutex as an option. Helen and Dr Ashton discuss this. Mark begins the day programme. He has strong feelings for one of the participants – he discusses it with Helen and Tony. He decides he needs a clearer head, that he needs to go for the Subutex, and detox. This is organised with the agreement of the day programme. Mark is to begin the Subutex the next Tuesday after taking his last methadone on the Monday.

CHAPTER 8

Treatment continues, preparing to move on

- Change of medication and community detoxification (Tier 3)
- Care co-ordination (Tier 3)
- Structured therapeutic counselling (Tier 3)
- Day programme (Tier 2)
- Liaison with other service provider out of area (Tier 2/3)
- Outreach/community support (Tier 2)

Monday 7 August – day programme
Mark attended and had a chat with Carrie and Brian during the coffee break about his planned switch to Subutex. 'It's good to know that's what is happening. If you find yourself needing to take time out from the group, that'll be OK, and someone can be with you. It's unlikely, but, you know, you won't be left alone with it.' Again they sought to reassure Mark.

> This consistency across services is so important. Different people saying different things is a menace to clients, particularly when they are facing something that they are likely to be anxious about. Mark's reassurance will be encouraged by this consistency.

The transition that Mark was going to undergo was raised in the group – with Mark's permission. Everyone was supportive and Mark felt a boost by that. The group also focused on what people's experiences had been over the weekend and whether the topics from last week had had any effect. There was a mixture of responses. Some people were still using and not really thinking much about their decision-making process, but others had been using the results of their work the previous Thursday. They all agreed that they were more mindful of overdose risks. During part of the afternoon, Brian and Carrie introduced some trust-building activities. They wanted to do this as the next phase was to help the participants to think about their own lives – to kind of do a life story, encourage them to be open about their experiences and experience receiving positive support from people through that reliving process.

Mark left and this time he was on the same bus as Mandy. He had arranged to meet up with a friend. He'd done that deliberately. He sat behind Mandy and they started chatting about the group, and how it was going. Mandy again suggested they continue the conversation at her place. Mark asked if she was planning to use – he didn't want to get into that. She said, 'no', she was trying to be more controlled in her use. They spent the rest of the day talking about their lives. Mark spent most of the time listening, Mandy did most of the talking. Shit, she'd had some bad times. Pretty much abandoned as a child, sexually abused by a neighbour, raped on numerous occasions, often under the influence of drugs. Mark knew it happened; he'd raped someone himself once under the influence, a situation that had got out of control. Hearing what Mandy was saying really left him feeling uncomfortable. He could feel that churning, spinning sensation inside himself again, and that weird numbness that had occurred in that last counselling session. He remembered what Tony had said, something about whether he could control the reactions.

He decided he'd better head home. Mandy burst into tears again when he suggested it and encouraged him to stay. He didn't leave until the next morning.

Meanwhile, Helen had phoned the drug service that served the area that Mark was going to. It was the local NHS service which she knew would be the one to take over from them once Mark moved. She needed to be sure they offered the services Mark needed, and if not, where they could be accessed. It turned out that they had similar Tier 3 services: care co-ordination, therapeutic counselling, and they had good links with the GPs, being keen to move people on into GP care once they were stable. Helen knew that so long as Mark could reduce and stop the Subutex that wouldn't be an issue, but it was interesting to her that they had this system well established – sounded a bit more so than their own. They were currently negotiating with their primary care trust to fund a similar set-up for 'shared care'.

Shared care is the system whereby the care of a client is shared between a GP and a substance misuse service. Often it will involve the GP prescribing for the client, for which they remain care co-ordinated from within the substance misuse team. It will involve regular feedback between professionals and three-way meetings at times to discuss progress and problems. Clients in shared care frequently are those who have stabilised to the degree that the GP – with support from the substance misuse service – feels able to prescribe. It has the advantage of keeping more stable clients away from substance misuse clinics where they are more likely to have contact with chaotic users, or those still dealing who may put them at risk of relapse. It frees up appointment slots in prescribing clinics for the more chaotic users, or those with more complex needs. It also ensures that a working relationship can be developed between the client and their GP. Shared care centres the healthcare provision with primary healthcare where there is access to a range of other healthcare services. Shared care also has an important educational role in encouraging GPs to take on prescribing responsibilities and deepen their understanding of substance misuse.

'So,' Helen continued in the conversation she was having with Dave who was the team leader, 'Mark expects to be coming down after his day programme ends. He's just starting the second week, and we hope to have him off the Subutex the week before.'

'That's fine. We can assess him here in terms of where he is at in himself when he gets down here. If you can send through your assessment for background.'

Open lines of communication and movement towards more standardised assessment helps ensure that information can flow for the benefit of clients.

'No problem, and I'll send a discharge letter as well, so you can see where things are the week he ends here. I think he'll need a fair bit of encouragement and support to begin with – not sure how he will be "drug-free". Big changes for him.'

'No, that's always an unknown. Some people adjust well, others just can't seem to get the idea of using again out of their heads for some time, and some never do. But we don't want to go back into maintenance prescribing if we can help it given what hopefully he will have achieved. We do have a community support worker down here; I'll let him know. He has the flexibility to spend time with people, and sort out any practical issues that come up.'

'Yeah. I wonder about him attending Narcotics Anonymous for support as well. Meet up with some people who have moved on, perhaps, and start to get to know a few people. I've kind of got mixed thoughts because it would leave him in touch with people who might still be using down with you, and I want him clear of all of that, but they can offer so much support.'

'Yeah, tough one to call. You going to mention it, or leave it until he gets down here?'

Helen thought about it. 'I'll mention it – maybe he could try a meeting or two up here and then he'll be in a more informed position to decide. At least then if he decides not to he won't have made contacts down with you that might bring him a bit too close to people who are still using. I don't know. You can't minimise the risk completely; life's a kind of risky business.'

'Yeah, our clients seem to have really internalised that one!'

'Anyway, I'll chat to him about it. It would be extra support for him, and I'll encourage him to think about it seriously and maybe give it a go.'

'Fine. So, you'll send the initial assessment and discharge letter – can we have the assessment now? We can allocate him to someone and they can be familiar with the background.'

'Sure, maybe get Mark to have a chat with him or her over the phone, perhaps, nearer the time of his moving down to you?'

'Sounds good. Anything to make the transition smooth and to reduce anxiety.'

'Yeah. Not sure how he's getting down. He must have stuff to take with him so ... Well, I don't know, something else to discuss with him.'

'Think he may come down to visit his ... who was it, his cousin?'

'Yeah, he may do that. Why?'

'Maybe he could drop in here if he's down during the week.'

'I'll mention that possibility if it comes up. I guess at the moment his week is pretty busy, but we can see if it arises.'

The conversation moved on to a general discussion about the work that the teams did, similarities and differences. It seemed that the team in Devon offered day programmes themselves, that the local Tier 2 service specialised in the outreach work as well as 'motivational interviewing' and social work interventions. They tended to pass on the more complex cases and it sounded like they had established good communication channels. They both agreed how crucial that was in order to make the Models of Care system work.

'How have you gone about ensuring training for Tier 1 and 2 staff in assessment? That's been a difficulty around here, people not wanting to get too involved, or in some instances, Tier 2 services trying to hang on to clients to boost their workload to keep their funding, rather than refer them on into Tier 3?'

'Yeah, was a problem but the managers got together and agreed to work together in seeking funding. There's a real sense of "joined-up" working around here. It's made a huge difference. By working collaboratively over funding issues it's taken out that competitive stuff that we all got saddled with during the bidding wars in the past.'

'Yeah, I've seen that happening as well, caused a lot of problems.'

'Well, we've got over all of that. You know, it really has become much more "client-centred", and less "service-centred". It really has freed people up in their attitudes. It's good. And we have inter-agency get-togethers as well, and not just at management level. That's a new thing that's recently been introduced. Getting everyone from services involved in drug and alcohol work – and some from Tier 1 services and the hospitals as well – to present on different themes and share in workshops. It really has made a big difference.'

'We're not there yet, but I'll pass it on because it sounds great.'

'Yeah, been too much division and budget protection in the past. Let's hope we've seen the last of that. Inter-agency working with clear, integrated care pathways – everyone clear what they offer to people on particular pathways – just made so much sense and, yes, it can work. But it does need working at. Like we said, communication.'

Helen was nodding as she listened to what Dave was saying. The clock caught her eye. She'd have to ring off soon; she had a client due in ten minutes and needed to get her paperwork done. She'd been taking notes during her conversation with Dave so she had the information for Mark.

'Look, I've got to go, but have you an info leaflet about the service you could send me?'

'Sure, I'll drop it in the post, and a few other bits and pieces about what we do.'

'Thanks, be good for Mark, but it's good for us to see how you present your services.'

'Yeah, maybe you can send me some stuff as well. No point in re-inventing wheels . . .'

'No probs. Yeah, that's a big one, seen a lot of that in the past as well . . . Anyway, thanks for all your help, and good luck with Mark. I hope we can send him down to you fit and ready for the next phase of his recovery.'

'Yeah, look forward to meeting him. Take care.'

'You too.'

Tuesday 8 August – switching over

Mark spent most of the day at the clinic. He began to experience withdrawal reactions mid-morning and they began the Subutex dosage, 6 mg to begin with. He went out a few times for some fresh air but generally stayed in throughout the day. The medication took him through the day. Yeah, he felt a little odd now and then, but he found having people to chat to sort of distracted him. He was still very aware of having spent the previous night with Mandy. Thank God he had some condoms with him – which reminded him, to get some more before he left at the end of the day. He was heading back to Mandy's. He wasn't sure what he was doing, but he felt he wanted to be with her.

He'd done a bit of work over the weekend for a friend – cash in hand. He was aware of actually having less money now he wasn't using. When he was on the gear he'd robbed to supplement his benefits, and usually had more than he needed, though it rarely seemed to get spent on food. Never could work out where it went. But he was having to think about his money now. He was planning a few more jobs here and there, and he knew he needed to get into work. He reckoned he'd find something once he'd moved.

Helen explained that Mark had enough buprenorphine in his system to take him through the night, and they would review him first thing in the morning. 'You might feel a withdrawal reaction by then but it shouldn't be too bad, given that we started you off today at 11.30am and you can be here 9.00am tomorrow.' Helen asked if he was alone that night, or whether Nick and Paula were around.

'I'm with a friend, I'll be OK.'

Helen checked out whether the friend was reliable. Mark nodded. He knew he had to be with Mandy but he didn't really want to say too much to Helen.

Wednesday 9 August – daily pick-up

Mark came in the next morning to pick up his next dose of medication. He said he'd been OK although he hadn't slept too well, was feeling tired now and a bit shaky and uncomfortable.

It was 9.30am when he took his medication for the day; the level was increased by 4 mg to 10 mg. They would review again the next day. He felt the Subutex kicking in and he was feeling a little more relaxed again and a bit light-headed, but not so doped up as he had done with the methadone. He had noticed that his thoughts had been racing a bit before he'd taken it. So many things he was having to think about.

He stayed for a while, then went for some fresh air. He had something to eat and came back and stayed at the clinic until his counselling session began. He was feeling OK. One of Helen's colleagues came and spoke to him for a while, asked how he was doing, took his blood pressure and pulse and was satisfied he was OK.

Counselling session
Tony was aware that Mark was switching medication. Helen had contacted him. He was grateful to know this. It would help him appreciate why there might be changes in Mark's behaviour. He made a point of letting Mark know at the start that Helen had told him. He asked how he was. Mark said he was OK so far.

Tony sensed that somehow Mark seemed pre-occupied, like he wasn't fully engaging with the process. He guessed it might be to do with the switch of medication, though he wasn't completely sure about that. He thought Subutex left people clearer, but then it was only the second day and there was a chemical adjustment taking place. Helen had said they increased the dose on the second day.

Mark didn't say much during the first part of the session; he found it difficult to engage with stuff about his past, or his future. He was stuck with what to do about Mandy.

Tony was becoming increasingly aware that something didn't feel right. He couldn't be clear what it was, but it was beginning to pre-occupy his thoughts and get in the way of his focus on Mark. He felt he needed to voice it and see if it had meaning for Mark. 'I'm sitting here with a sense that something's wrong, or difficult, or something, Mark, I don't know what it is and I don't want to push you, but I want to make what I'm feeling here visible.'

Mark stayed silent. He took a deep breath, held it, and then let it out. He didn't know what to say. He knew that the counselling was confidential, but he knew that Tony had said there were limits to this, particularly if he was threatening or behaving in ways that would put him or others at risk. Did that include him messing around with his medication? He'd used some methadone the previous evening. Mandy'd got it. Seemed like a good idea at the time. But it had left him feeling really bad in the night, though it had passed. He knew he shouldn't have done it, and he wanted to talk about it, he knew he had to, but would it go any further? He was worried he might do it again, but didn't feel he could talk to Helen in case they put him back on the methadone again, which he knew he didn't want to have happen. He didn't know. Would Tony talk to Helen? He didn't want to mess everything up. He knew that they were trying to help. Fuck it, he thought, why didn't I listen to what I was being told last week? I shouldn't have got involved.

The silence continued. Tony could sense Mark's discomfort. He clearly had something on his mind, but wasn't saying it. Tony decided his empathic sensitivity was justification for enquiring. 'What is it, Mark? What's happened?'

Mark shook his head. 'I'm not sure I can say.'

'Something you don't want me to know?'

Mark sighed. 'I'm not sure how confidential it is here.'

'Something you don't want me to pass on?'

Mark nodded.

'OK, well if you're going to tell me you're planning to harm yourself or someone else then, yes, I have to pass that on. Is that what it's about?'

'Not exactly.'

'OK, not exactly harm to yourself or someone else, but ...'

'I've got a problem.' Mark was clearly struggling to say what was on his mind.

Tony sensed the difficulty and decided that maybe, if Mark needed to talk something out, then perhaps the answer was to keep it hypothetical and see how it developed. 'Let's suppose we keep it hypothetical, like as if you're talking about someone else?'

'Like me having a friend that has done something?'

'Yeah.'

> What does another professional do with this kind of information? It should depend on what has been agreed locally – what protocols are in place for disclosure of this kind. And yet, if they are too tight and explicit, clients may not divulge this information and as a result put themselves and others at greater risk. By introducing the hypothetical style, Tony has encouraged Mark to talk.

'OK, it's like, what would you do if someone, a friend, yeah, who used something as well as his medication, when he wasn't supposed to, and, well, might do it again. I mean, what would you do with that information?'

'I suppose it would depend whether it was putting that someone at risk and whether it was likely to be repeated.'

Mark nodded. 'It won't be repeated. I know I can't do it again.'

Tony noted the shift into the first person. 'So, you won't do it again, but it's on your mind, yeah?'

'Yeah. Oh fuck, this is stupid, I've got to say and sort it out. I used methadone last night, stupid thing to do, felt fucking awful, some kind of a reaction, but if Helen or Dr Ashton knew, they might, I don't know, stop the medication, put me back on methadone again, or something, and I really don't want that. I fucked up, Tony, and I want to see Mandy but I can't, can I?'

'Two dilemmas: who do you tell, and what do you do about Mandy?' Tony was aware that Mark had not mentioned Mandy.

'I can't go back to her again today, I know that, it would be stupid.' She was bad news, he didn't need it. But the pull to be with her was still there. The sex had been fucking good – well, good fucking. He hadn't realised he was smiling to himself.

Tony noted the smile. 'Good thoughts?'

'Mhmm? Yeah.' The smile faded as he came back to his dilemma. He took a deep breath and started to tell Tony what had happened, at least his being with Mandy and that, well, he couldn't go back to her and risk it happening again, and he really hoped Tony wasn't going to say anything.

'I can appreciate the difficulty, Mark, and I want to say that I think Helen needs to know what has happened. And maybe if you can tell her and reassure her that you're not going to be with Mandy again, but go back to where you were with your friends. I don't know what effect the methadone use will have had, and whether it means that you may need more Subutex, or what, but I do advise you to talk to her.'

Mark isn't really listening, more in touch with his sense of always fucking up. At least, though, this can now be explored. It is probably a huge belief system that Mark is carrying and which will need dealing with as he seeks sustainable change and greater self-belief.

Mark was silent, and Tony felt the atmosphere change. 'I always fuck up – story of my life.'

'That how it feels, yeah, fuck everything up, huh?'

'What's the point? None of it'll work out, will it? I mean, something'll happen. I'll end up using again. I'm a fucking addict, aren't I? I hate it, but that's me, who I am, what I am!' He was raising his voice. 'Fuck it, fuck everything.'

Tony stayed with him and with the rising anger. He sensed that while it was being released in the context of his feelings about himself, maybe it had its roots way back and it needed to come out.

'Yeah, fuck it all.' Tony waited.

Mark could feel himself getting more angry with himself, but not just himself, with everything, everyone. The bastard Eric's face appeared in his head. He wanted to smash him. Hadn't seen him now for years, but he knew he'd never forgive him for what had happened in the past. His jaw had tightened and he could feel his heart pounding. His face felt like it was glowing, but none of it stood out against the boiling anger he was feeling. He tightened his fists and looked up, then tried to release them, but the tightness was still there. He held his fists in front of him. He wanted to punch something, and punch it hard. 'Fuck it!' The words exploded out of his mouth and he slammed both his fists down on the arms of the chair. He closed his eyes; he wasn't trying to compose himself, or regain control, he wasn't there. He felt so full of energy; he got up and paced around, starting to punch his right fist into his left hand.

'The anger's really in your body, Mark, bubbling and boiling away.'

Mark heard him and he thought, yeah, too bloody right, but he didn't say anything, just carried on punching his fist into his hand. He leant back against the wall, tightly closing his eyes while he clasped his fist. Tony could see the fingers of his left hand turning white. So much tension.

Tony stayed calm. He wasn't going to get over-excited or start panicking. Yeah, Mark was angry and he was burning up with it. And that was probably a good thing. He hadn't made to start breaking up the room or anything – and anyway, sometimes that was necessary though he would always try to help clients avoid that where possible.

'I want to hit something, I want to hit something hard, something really hard.'

Tony noted the thickness of the chair cushion. 'Here, take this, put it against the wall, or on the floor and let it have it, preferably the outside wall here, it's solid.'

Mark took the cushion and battered it with the side of his fist. It wasn't enough; he needed both fists. He threw it on to the floor and let fly at it. 'Fuck it, fuck it, fuck it.'

Tony sat leaning forward, keeping his attention on Mark and being open to his feeling of compassion for this guy, so tormented with anger, desperate for change, but at the same time risking sabotaging it all. Yeah, he'd every right to feel angry, and no doubt his past was all caught up in it as well.

'Fucking bastard.' Mark took another thump at the cushion.

'Yeah, fucking bastard.' He didn't ask who it was, just stayed being in empathic touch with what was happening through Mark's words.

'If he hadn't buggered off . . . but it wouldn't have been any different. Still been a fucking nightmare. Just wouldn't have had the other fucker coming into my home.'

'Your father, yeah?'

Mark nodded. 'Yeah, and Eric.'

'Two men.' As Tony said it he was wondering where it had come from and was making a note to talk it through in supervision. He was directing the focus onto gender and it wasn't where Mark was appearing to have his focus.

'But it wasn't really them, I mean, it was that bitch of a mother. All that seemed to matter was her drugs. I mean, she did care for us – sort of. Never had social services coming through the door – maybe we should have had – but it was, what, 15 years ago. Just a fucking nightmare.'

'Yeah, fucking nightmare, and still in your head, yeah?'

Mark nodded. He was suddenly feeling very tired. His hands were sore, particularly the sides down to his wrists where he'd been slamming into the cushion.

'You must think I'm mad.'

'No. Angry, and maybe other feelings as well, but not mad.'

'I feel better for that.' Mark was getting up and putting the cushion back in the chair.

'Good. Got something out of the system, yeah?'

'Yeah, still bloody angry with myself over this Mandy thing, though. Think I should come clean?'

'What do you think?'

'Bloody scary, like, I'm losing control.'

'Losing control?'

'Over what happens next.'

'Mhmm. Control's important?'

'Too much time not in control. Yeah, I like to be in control, but I tell Helen and, fuck, the shit's really in the fan.'

'Tough one to call.'

Mark had slumped down in the chair. 'I'm not going back to Mandy. I'm heading back to Nick and Paula. I mean, they can be a bit crazy at times, but they're who I need to be with.'

'They sound important to you.'

'Yeah. They're supportive. They want to see me move on, get myself together. They've been through it, and they have difficult times, but they care, you know, I mean, yeah, I'll go back there. No more Mandy.'

'You sound like you've made a clear decision.'

'Yeah, and I'm going to learn from it. I'm too vulnerable at the moment, too all over the place. I need my focus. I need to be clear about my goals here.' He was shaking his head again. 'But I'm afraid I'll fuck up somehow. I mean, that's really scary.'

'Fear of fucking up, yeah? It all means so much to you to keep your focus.'

Is it unprofessional to mirror a client's use of language in this way? Perhaps for some professions, but for the counsellor it is about engaging with the client, conveying back what they have heard and what they understand from what the client is communicating. Sometimes it is necessary to swear like this in order to convey this sense of appreciation for what the client is experiencing. For the client, there is a real fear of what he describes as becoming 'fucked up'. The counsellor conveys that he has heard this. Having felt heard, the client now moves on to talk about something else. Another response could have been to encourage the client to describe what he meant from what he had said. That would also have been helpful, but this is not the line this particular counsellor takes.

'I need to be thinking about the future, making sure it happens. Helen's talking to the service down in Devon, making sure it'll all be smooth when I go. I'm really grateful for that. And what do I do?' He stared down at the floor and sighed. He looked up and into Tony's eyes. 'I need to be straight with her, don't I?'

'That's what you're feeling, yeah?'

'Yeah. Shit, that's scary.'

They both sat in silence: Mark trying to imagine how Helen would react, what would happen, and feeling sorry and stupid; Tony holding in his awareness his sense of Mark's scared feeling.

Time was passing and the session was soon due to end. Tony mentioned the time.

'OK. I'll tell Helen. It is best.'

Tony wanted to trust Mark. He felt it therapeutically important to do so, and he acknowledged to himself his sense of Mark's genuineness in what he was saying.

'OK. I'm sure she'll appreciate you being open about it, and she'll know that you could have said nothing and she'd be none the wiser. But she's obviously going to insist it doesn't happen again ...' Tony was aware that he was reassuring Mark about things that he couldn't guarantee. He recognised that he probably wanted Mark to say something and was relieved that he was planning to.

Mark left and headed back to Nick and Paula's. He later phoned Mandy to say he wasn't coming over, had things to do, and wasn't sure that being with her was actually helping him. She got angry, saying he'd used her. He genuinely didn't feel that he had; in fact, he felt used himself. He had to put the phone down. He hadn't given her his number, and he'd had his brain in gear enough to hold back the number when he dialled. Of course, he knew he'd have to see her at the group the next day. He was feeling edgy, anxious. Had a can of lager. Knew he shouldn't but he needed it. Felt calmed down a bit and it took him through the evening. Spent time talking to Nick and Paula about the situation. Watched a bit of TV and then headed to bed. Couldn't sleep. By 2.00am he'd had enough and had another can. He eventually fell asleep. He slept fitfully. He overslept.

The next few weeks
Mark continued to attend the group, and the counselling, and successfully reduced down his Subutex. He told Helen what had happened the next morning and made it clear it wasn't going to happen again. Helen made it clear that if it did, he'd be back on supervised methadone consumption again. Dr Ashton wasn't happy either, and Mark got another lecture from him. He stressed that trust was all important. They needed him to stick to the regime. They kept him under review. Mark stabilised and they agreed that they'd begin the gradual withdrawal the next Monday. They re-assigned Phil, the outreach worker, to spend time with him during the week when he wasn't at the programme. In fact, he met up with Phil two or three times during the week, sometimes for a coffee after the programme.

He was reduced down 2 mg at a time, four days at the next level, then reduce again. So after 16 days he was on 2 mg and looking at the final drop down to nothing – the biggest step of all. His smoking of tobacco had increased.

> An interesting point to consider is around how often drug services address tobacco. It is the biggest killer drug and yet it is accepted that people can use tobacco to compensate, to help them quell anxiety. Should all substances be integrated into substance misuse services? If so, at what level of use does one define smoking as problematic?

His drinking had also gone up, not dramatically, but there was an increase. Mark was still defensive about this, not seeing it as a problem. Didn't feel his two cans of an evening was a problem, well, yes, sometimes he had four, but only sometimes. Previously he hadn't been drinking every day. Both Helen and Dr Ashton had explained the dangers of substituting one substance for another, but Mark was insistent that he would be OK. They decided to keep on with the reduction regime. At least Mark was drinking mid-range beers – 4% to 5%, eight to ten units maximum per day so he wasn't going to be alcohol-affected 24/7. They knew though that he'd need to monitor his alcohol use once he was off the Sub-utex and they'd need to make the service in Devon aware of this.

Mandy's using had increased the moment Mark said he wasn't coming round any more, and she lost interest in the group. She didn't turn up to the next session. When she came the following week – somewhat drug-affected – it all blew up in the group. She threatened to tell the facilitators he'd used methadone on top. Mark countered it by telling them himself, and pointed out that he had told Helen, but that they could check with her, and that he wasn't going to do it again, he'd learned a tough lesson. In fact, the result of it all was that Mandy dropped out of the programme. Carrie discussed with Helen as to whether Mark should leave as well; however, they hadn't made 'no sexual relationship with other participants' a ground rule for the group, having merely pointed out that it was not advisable.

The programme moved on to address the participants' life stories. Mark had found it hard to write. His first attempt was too short and he was encouraged to have another go. It was very emotional. It was a four-can session the evening afterwards – took him a while to settle down.

Helen had received the information about services in North Devon from Dave. It made interesting reading. They had developed some ideas that were new to her. One was about user groups. They'd had a user group for a while, but it wasn't well attended – clients sometimes saying it was a waste of time. Everyone who had facilitated it over the years had struggled with it as well. But Dave's service had something they called a community meeting. Once a month they stopped services for a couple of hours and made the clinic 'open house', so to speak, and had a session in which any and all clients could attend, and all staff were also expected to attend. It was minuted, action points were established, and there was feedback on these action points at the next meeting. While there was an agenda, the tone of the meeting was very informal. Dave had included a brief report on it. Helen thought it sounded good. She liked the idea of everyone getting together like that, and she also liked the idea of calling it a 'community meeting' – that somehow sounded more level, more inclusive, than 'user group' which still carried a strong element of labelling. She was determined to push the idea with the team. They had a large room they could use.

She also noted that, like many other services, they used acupuncture, but not just auricular acupuncture for relaxation and detoxification. They'd got funding for a fully trained acupuncturist to work with clients who wanted it, extending the breadth of the treatment, helping to rebalance the client's energy system. It had proved popular. They also had aromatherapy sessions as well. Helen had looked into this herself some while back but there hadn't been funding. They had tried to get volunteers to offer a service, but that had drawn a blank. What she read fired her enthusiasm once more and she spoke to the team leader about it.

In spite of national standards there will always be scope for regional and local variation. Some services do attract interest in one area, and not in others. The provision of complementary therapy is an example of this. Many services use this and to good effect. Others do not. Some clients value it, wanting alternatives to drug responses to drug problems. Some teams offer it to engage with clients. Often auricular acupuncture is used for detoxification. Others argue that fully trained acupuncturists should be working with clients to work with their whole system, not just for a specific treatment, thereby ensuring a more holistic intervention. The mass of practice-based evidence should be drawn together nationally so that informed choices can be made.

Friday 25 August – prescribing clinic
Mark was now down to 2 mg, and it was time to reduce again; however, both Dr Ashton and Helen felt that he should maybe stay on the 2 mg over the weekend and then reduce the following Monday when he had access to support. Mark was keen to finally kick it, but he could see the sense in what they were saying. His life had changed a lot. He was clearer in himself now, much clearer. He'd had some tough counselling sessions, he was much more aware of his feelings and still trying to come to terms with them. He still had anger about his past, and increasing amounts of sadness would bubble through as well. They'd looked at the losses they had had on the day programme, and it was awesome how much loss everyone had experienced. It was a tough day for everyone. Just seeing all your losses laid out, kind of end to end, throughout your life. Yeah, left him feeling sad, or maybe, more accurately, more in touch with sadness he'd been carrying for years but using to keep away from.

He was feeling more alive but that didn't mean feeling more comfortable, but he had grown to accept that. Having Phil meeting up with him outside of the clinic had really helped. Spending time chatting, and not just about his programme or the drugs, was great. And he was all geared up for the move, he thought to himself. He smiled. 'Geared up', that would have meant something quite different a few weeks back! But that was history, and he had to make sure it stayed that way.

He had two more weeks of the programme to do, and he had made arrangements with his cousin about going down the weekend after that final week. He was now keen to get away although he was also aware of feeling uncomfortable about leaving. He knew it would be strange, but he had to get on with his life.

Thursday 31 August
The day programme had been good and Mark was sitting with Phil having a chat. Mark was now four days into being clean and it had been difficult. Anxieties had risen to the surface. He was aware of his own sensitivity even more. Somehow that last 2 mg jump seemed huge. He was talking to Phil about it.

'Yeah, it's like jumping from something to nothing, which can feel a lot bigger than something to something less.'

'And it's knowing that's it, no more. Kind of brings on the memories and that's not easy.'

'What, times you've used?'

Mark nodded. 'Spent most of the counselling session on Wednesday reminiscing.'

'So, how do you feel about it all now, looking back, knowing that's it, you're heading in another direction?'

Mark didn't hesitate. 'Feels good, feels scary.'

Phil nodded. 'Yeah, and you're doing well. And you'll get more support when you've moved and the sun and sand, yeah, sounds like you're heading for a good life, Mark.'

Mark smiled. He certainly hoped so. He knew he couldn't stay around. His mum had reacted badly to his saying he was going. He'd held back from telling her, but had done so now. Her reaction made him more determined to go, though as well he did feel sorry for her, well, it was more pity than anything else. Yeah, he wanted to help her, but they always argued and she really wasn't there for him, more concerned about her needs, how she would cope. That's all she talked about. He needed to be away.

Friday 1 September – prescribing clinic
'You're doing well, Mark, really well.' Dr Ashton was pleased that Mark was hold-ing his abstinence. He was not going to stop seeing him simply because he was off the Subutex and not using. He wanted to maintain continuity for Mark until he moved on, and so he could send a letter himself about his progress on to the doctor at the other drug and alcohol service. They took a final blood test. They'd have the result the next week and the details of that could also be sent on.

'Thanks.'

'So, what are your plans?'

'Well, I'm going to help Rod for a while, he's got a removal business. That'll be hard work, I know, but it'll keep me busy, get me fit and, yeah, get me some money. I really want to work in this area later, you know? I've talked to a lot of people here and, yeah, I'd like to be part of something like this one day.'

'Mhmm, many people who used drugs in the past do that, Mark, but you need to have a while to be clear of it all. Some people get involved too quickly and they can lose it.'

'How long?'

'Couple of years. Really get yourself established and then see. People are moti-vated for all kinds of reasons, sometimes these are healthy reasons – wanting to help others, you know? But sometimes it is about wanting to belong to some-thing – like a substitute family.'

Mark took a deep breath. 'Yeah, funny you should say that, but this place has been like a family to me; at times I feel like I've moved in! You've kind of accepted me in, even though I did stupid things at the start which could have meant you'd throw me out.'

'We try to avoid that, if we sense someone is really serious. When someone is simply messing us about, then we may need to look at other arrangements. But we're here to reduce or minimise harm, not contribute to situations where a person is at more risk. Like when you used on top, or you gave some of your med-ication away, yeah, it happens. But we don't want to lose contact with people over it if we can avoid it, but we also have to ensure that people are medically safe, you know?'

'Yeah. Overdosing, lot of it about.'

'Yes, but not much round here, fortunately; we try to keep our prescribing tight and contained, hence the supervised consumption.'

The session drew to a close with more encouraging words from Dr Ashton. Mark then spent a while with Helen. She offered him the opportunity to talk about anything on his mind, aware that Mark was passing through a lot of endings at the moment which would feel like losses – the day programme, the people on it, Tony, Phil, herself, Dr Ashton – people who had all been important for Mark in his progress in recent weeks. Plus leaving the area, his friends. She'd spoken again to Dave about Mark being seen early when he moved down there. They'd given her an appointment for him and were sending a letter. It would be on the Wednesday the week after he moved down. 'Give him a couple of days to settle in, get himself a GP and stuff.' He'd mentioned one of the surgeries in the area where they had good liaison links. 'Hopefully, it won't be a problem, but it makes sense for him to register there.'

They also arranged for Mark's new care co-ordinator, Lizzie, to phone him while he was at the clinic, have a quick chat, hopefully ease any anxieties around stepping into the unknown. Helen told Mark of this and gave him the other information Dave had given her verbally about his appointment. Mark told her how he was feeling in limbo at the moment. He was thinking ahead although he couldn't really imagine it – it would be so different, and yet he didn't really feel such a part of things here, now. Like something had moved inside him. He knew the next week would be tough, seeing everyone for the last time. Asked if he could have a longer session next Friday in case he needed it.

'Sure, I think we need time to process endings not only when we are preparing for them, but as they are happening. And, of course, you won't really know what it is like – the actual moving on – until it has happened.'

Mark nodded. 'And that's what's weird, like, something is going to happen, it's inevitable, it's out there just a week away now, and yet I can't really imagine it, not really. Any changes in the past, well, I've always been drug-affected, you know, but this is so different, so new.'

The phone rang; it was Lizzie. Helen gave Mark the phone and left the room, said she'd be back when he finished the call.

'Hi Mark, so you're coming down to us. You'll enjoy it down here.'

'I've visited my cousin and, yeah, I like the area.'

Lizzie kept the conversation informal for a bit longer, hoping to make it feel easy for Mark.

'So, I'm seeing you on the Wednesday, yeah, 13 September, 10.00am. We've put a map of how to find us in with the letter that should be with you any time now.'

'Thanks.'

'And we understand you want to carry on with some therapeutic counselling for a while?'

Mark said he was, that it had been helpful but he was aware of how much adjustment he was having to make, and he was still feeling sensitive about a lot of things in his life, and feeling he could work at it, keep up the momentum so to speak, would be good. Lizzie confirmed that they were organising this, that there'd be a short wait until one of their counsellors had a free space, but shouldn't be more than a couple of weeks.

Mark was reassured as much by Lizzie's tone as what she was saying. And she had quite a local accent as well. Somehow that made her sound more welcoming. She also mentioned about his need to register with a GP when he got down and mentioned the surgery they had particularly good links with. Mark agreed to sort that before his appointment with her.

The conversation drew to a close, and Lizzie rang off. Yeah, it felt good to have spoken to her. Somehow it would have felt kind of harder not knowing who or what he was heading to. He felt reassured. It made a difference. Little thing, a few minutes on the phone, but yeah, somehow it helped to bring his future into the present. He really was moving on; he really *was* moving on, he thought to himself.

He opened the door to see if Helen was around.

'Finished, then, all go OK?'

Mark nodded. 'Yeah, she sounded nice, told me a bit about the place and confirmed my appointment and that they were organising therapeutic counselling for me.' He shook his head. 'Brought it all closer, somehow, talking to her like that.'

Helen smiled. 'Yes, and I think it's important, part of the transition process. By the way, how're you moving down?'

'Rod's removal business – haven't got much, but he's coming up in one of their smaller vans. Got clothes, stereo, TV, few books, bits and pieces, you know? More than I could take on the train. Yeah, it's all organised. Saturday morning. Going out for a meal with Nick and Paula on Friday night.'

'Not seeing your mother?'

Mark shook his head. 'I can't. What's the point? She'll make it harder for me, I know she will. I've got to move on. I'll keep in touch with her, yeah, and once I'm settled I'll come back to visit, but not now, not at the moment.'

Mark looked sad. Helen mentioned it.

Mark nodded. 'Yeah. I mean, you know, she brought me into the world, and yeah, maybe now I'm feeling more grateful for that, now that I feel I've got a future, you know? But she does my head in, I need space, normality, be with normal people, you know, who don't run to drugs to cope. Normality, and a bit of peace, yeah, chill out a bit. But yeah, just – I say be normal, but I'm not sure what that means.'

'I guess it's about becoming who you are, realising more of your own potential, you know? I mean, you've got to know yourself better these past few weeks, and you've changed, yeah? That'll continue, no doubt.'

He took a deep breath. 'Yeah and I do want to get into this kind of work. I'm thinking of training in counselling myself, go along to an introductory course or something; there are some around. I expect there'll be something down there.'

'Good way to start, get a feel for it, see what it's like, an opportunity to experience yourself in another world, so to speak.'

Mark smiled. 'Done a lot of that in the past. Now comes the real world, a world you don't use drugs to get into, only to get out of!'

Helen smiled. 'Nice one-liner. Mind if I use it?'

'Feel free.'

'Keep it together, Mark, keep your focus, and you'll get there.'

That felt good to hear. He hoped so, he really hoped so.

Summary

Helen contacts the substance misuse team in Devon, and they arrange for a transfer of information. They decide to give Mark a community care worker at the start and refer him for further counselling as well as provide him with a care co-ordinator. Mark begins the switch to buprenorphine, spends a couple of nights with Mandy, and uses methadone with her. He realises he's been stupid, which leads him to connect with and release pent-up anger from his past within the counselling session. He detoxes over a few weeks, anger and increasing sadness rising to the surface. He gets support from the outreach worker. His mother is making it difficult for him, reacting badly to his decision to move away. Mark speaks over the phone to Lizzie, his new care co-ordinator in Devon.

CHAPTER 9

Endings, suicide attempt and a new beginning?

- Prescribing clinic post-detoxification (Tier 3)
- Care co-ordination (Tier 3)
- Structured therapeutic counselling (Tier 3)
- Day programme (Tier 2)
- Outreach/community support (Tier 2)

Future: following referral to new service

- Care co-ordination (Tier 3)
- Structured therapeutic counselling (Tier 3)
- Relapse prevention group (Tier 2)

Wednesday 6 September – counselling session

Mark attended the session; it was his last one. Tony was on holiday the following week and so this was the first of Mark's goodbyes. He'd really come to appreciate Tony, his style, his way of being; he always seemed to be there, listening, taking him seriously, caring. It was something new to him, never really telling him what to do, and yet somehow he seemed to convey a kind of wisdom, a sort of calm assurance. He'd come to look forward to the sessions even though they had been tough going at times. He had grown to appreciate the contrasting styles as well. Helen was practical, down to earth, concerned, always ready to try to make things happen for him. She sort of bustled him along and he needed that. Meanwhile Tony gave him a more reflective space, and that was valuable too. Yeah, he could see the value in the two different ways of working.

Part of the session was given over to conveying to each other what they had appreciated about the work they had done together. For Tony it was the determination that Mark had shown in spite of difficulties. He'd started out not sure what counselling was about and where it would take him, but he had used it and grown through it. Yes, there was more for him to do; the past still left his head in confusion. He still had to develop a clear sense of himself as a non-drug-dependent person. But that would come as he cultivated a new lifestyle and his sense of self developed in parallel. He was glad Mark was going to continue the counselling and he hoped that he would go the distance.

It was hard for Mark to go. He actually felt quite emotional. So did Tony, who was never one to hide his emotions when they were present and related to his client. They both had tears in their eyes and lumps in their throats as they hugged.

'So, you take care of yourself, Mark, you're doing well, you're going to learn a lot about yourself, and when you become a counsellor,' Mark had mentioned this in one of the sessions, 'I'm sure you'll be a good one. You have a lot of natural sensitivity – but it got buried with the drugs – and you have an appreciation of the struggle people go through, and how far-reaching change has to be. Yeah, I wish you well. Get yourself together and get out there and make a difference.'

Mark smiled; he really did have a big lump in his throat now. He closed his eyes and nodded his head. 'Thanks for that. It's what I want. It's my goal. It'll take time. I've got to get used to working at something and not expecting everything to be instant. I've learned that now. Thanks for everything, Tony, thanks.' Tony followed him out to the waiting area.

'Bye.'

'Thanks again. Bye.'

Monday 11 September
The telephone rang and Carrie picked it up.

'Hi, Carrie, it's Mark. Look, something's come up and I'm not going to make it today, I'm really sorry.'

'Can you tell me what's happened, Mark? I'm sorry you won't be able to make it.'

'It's my mum. She's overdosed. In hospital. On tubes and all kinds of stuff. It's all touch and go. She really went for it. God knows what she's done to herself.'

'So are you at the hospital?'

'Yeah. Came up last night. She's still unconscious. I'd arranged to go around to see her Sunday evening. She'd taken paracetamol – bloody stuff, and a bottle of vodka. It was planned, getting at me for going. I want to say fucking bitch, and yet, well, she's my mum. Seeing her all tubed up in here – oh fuck, this is all I need.'

Carrie knew about Mark's plans. His last week in the area. Shit, she thought, how fucking devious can you get? Either his mum is so desperate for him to be there, or it's revenge or ... she couldn't understand it, but she knew this kind of thing happened.

'Have you told Helen?'

'No. Thought I'd best call here first.'

'Do you want to call her or shall I let her know?'

'Don't know. I don't know. Don't know what to do, Carrie, don't know what to do.'

'Are you on your own?'

'Yeah. My brother Trev I couldn't contact – he must be away somewhere. So, yeah, just me.'

'Look, let me call Helen. Maybe you need someone with you, Mark, would that help?'

'I don't know. I just . . . I don't know.'

Carrie knew this was going to be a hugely high-risk time for Mark, but she wasn't going to bring up drugs. He was in crisis and he needed support. She decided the best thing was to take control of the situation.

'Mark, I'll get a message to Helen. Which hospital are you at?'

'The General.'

'OK. I'll tell Helen.'

'Thanks. I guess I'd better go back. Just seem to be drinking coffee at the moment. Didn't sleep much last night. I want to get away from it all, Carrie, and I know that I don't, but I do. I don't feel safe.'

'Yeah.' She saw Brian walking past the doorway. She called out to him and he came in. 'I've got Mark on the phone, his mum has overdosed badly, unconscious, in the General, Mark's there. He's in a mess. Can you call Helen? I'll carry on talking to him. I think someone needs to go over there, maybe one of their outreach people, someone, anyone. He's on his own with it. We need to get containment if we can.'

'OK.' Brian went off to call Helen; he explained what had happened. She was expecting a booked client any moment, so she called Phil on his mobile. He was about to go out on a used needle collection run. She explained what had happened. He said he'd head straight over to the hospital. Poor bugger. He'd lost his mum a couple of years back, nothing this dramatic, but one hell of a shock all the same. He diverted to the hospital.

'My client's arrived. Phil, can you call the day programme and let them know you're on your way? They're still talking to Mark on the phone.'

'Sure, give me their number.'

Phil phoned and got Brian. Carrie was still talking to Mark. 'Hi, Phil, outreach?'

'Hi, yeah, Brian here.'

'I'm heading to the hospital now. Is Carrie still on the line with Mark?'

'Yeah, I think so.'

'Let him know I'll be with him in hopefully about 20 minutes, depending on traffic. Bad time of day.'

'Yeah, sure, will do.'

Meanwhile, Carrie was checking out with Mark if he was OK with her saying what had happened to the group by way of explaining why he was not there, or to simply say that something had come up.

'No, tell them. We've been learning about being real. Can't change that now.'

'Sure?'

'Yeah.'

'OK.'

Brian called over to Carrie. 'Phil's heading over to the hospital – be there in 20 minutes or so depending on traffic.'

'Brian's just told me Phil is heading over to be there with you, be 20 minutes or so, depending on traffic.'

Mark felt a sudden sense of relief. He liked Phil. Yeah, he was glad it was him. 'Thanks for organising that. You people, you're like diamonds. Thanks. Look, I'd better get back and see what's happening. I'll be there on Thursday, I promise.'

'Sure, and we'll look forward to seeing you, Mark. Take it easy. I know it's a tough time, but take it easy.'

'Yeah. Thanks.' He hung up.

In moments of crisis, inter-agency co-operation can be vital in ensuring that a crisis gets managed as opposed to being left 'for someone else to deal with', and the result is a client at best using to cope temporarily and at worse plunging back into old patterns of use. Two crucial elements of the Models of Care system are communication and clarity of role and responsibility. Here we see an example of two teams working together, drawing in people to respond to the need that has arisen. Teams need flexibility and staff provision to allow this. Crisis happens for clients of substance misuse services. There needs to be staff capacity to respond.

Carrie and Brian told the group and it sort of set the tone for the rest of the morning. Set off a discussion around relationships with parents, coping with sudden problems, all kinds of issues. Judy said she was going to get him a card at lunch time and they could all sign it. Everyone felt good about that. The general feeling was that one of their group, their family, was missing, having a tough time. They wanted to show they were thinking about him, missing him, hoping all would be well.

Phil arrived at the hospital. He was slightly later than he expected – nowhere to park. He'd managed to find the intensive care section and the waiting area. No sign of Mark. He asked at the reception, said he was a friend come over to offer support. Mark was in the room with his mum; she had woken up but wasn't able to say anything, and was drifting in and out of sleep. Phil went over and found them.

'Hi.' He tightened his lips. There wasn't much to say, really, the situation spoke for itself.

'Hi Phil. Thanks for coming over. She's woken up but is still out of it.'

'How're you doing?'

Mark shrugged.

'Want to come away for a chat – what's best for you?'

'Yeah. At least she's awake now.'

They went outside; Mark wanted to smoke.

'Bugger, isn't it?'

'Yeah. Not surprised but, well . . .'

Phil nodded.

'So you're kind of on your own with it?'

'Yeah, couldn't get in touch with my brother, he's away, so, yeah.' He shook his head. 'What the fuck do I do now?'

'Why'd she do it?'

'Get at me – has to be that. She'd set it up, invited me over, knew when I was coming, and had just downed the paracetamol and the vodka and waited for me to arrive.'

'Dangerous game. You could have been delayed.'

'Yeah. And that would have been that. Doctors are still very concerned about how much damage she's done to her liver. Seems as though it's bad but they're doing tests.'

'Timed to perfection, huh?'

Mark shook his head. 'Yeah.'

'And I guess you've got so many different feelings running around at the moment . . .'

'I don't know whether to be sad or angry. I actually think I feel more angry, you know, and part of me wishes I'd not gone round now. Is that so awful? But that's how I feel. I'd be better off without her.' He took a deep breath. 'But she's my mum and what the hell do I do?' He was shaking his head again.

'Yeah.'

They both lapsed into silence. Mark took a deep drag on his cigarette.

'So I guess I'm not heading down to Devon now.'

'You said that with a heavy heart.'

Mark nodded slowly as he took another deep breath. 'I know I need to get away, but, I don't know.'

'What difference could you make if you stayed?' Phil could feel himself wanting to encourage Mark to go, stick to his plans, not get dragged back into the emotional blackmail that was clearly going on.

'I dunno really. Feel I guess I ought to. Feel it's all my fault.'

'Your fault, that you were hoping for a better life, a fresh start, an opportunity for change?'

'Yeah, well, something always happens, doesn't it. Everything always fucks up on me.'

Phil wanted to confront him but he didn't want to push him; it was all too sensitive, too close. He knew that others in the team would be talking to Mark and he guessed that probably the general feeling was likely to be that he needed to make the move although he could still come back and visit if he wanted to. What a tough call, though.

'Sometimes we can still turn it around. Don't make any sudden changes of plan, Mark, give it some thought. Think about what it'll be like if you stay, and how it could be if you stick to your plans.'

'Yeah. I know, she's being fucking manipulative.'

'Yeah, and she's probably scared about you going, for her own reasons. She can't see the advantages for you, only the loss for her.'

'Don't see why it's a loss for her; she hasn't given much of a toss for me most of my life.'

Phil didn't reply, rather allowing what Mark had said to stay with him.

Mark had finished his cigarette. 'I need another coffee.'

'OK, let's go to the coffee shop here, or do you want to go around the corner? There are a couple of places there.'

'Let's get out of here. Place gives me the creeps.'

They headed round the corner to a café.

'Have you eaten anything today?'

'No.'

'How about a breakfast, give you some energy.'

'Ought to eat but I don't fancy it.'

'Clinic'll pay.' Phil guessed it might be a money decision. 'Compared to the cost of the medication we dish out, one breakfast isn't going to break the bank, and probably do more for you at the moment!'

'OK, I'll give it a go.'

They chatted while they waited for the food to arrive. His mobile went off; it was Helen. 'How're things, Phil?'

He explained what they were doing.

'Does Mark want to come over to the clinic later for a chat?'

He asked him. Said he wasn't sure what he was going to do. Phil gave him the phone.

'Feel free to come over, Mark. I'm around most of the afternoon catching up on some admin. And we've the appointment tomorrow.'

'Yeah. I'll see how it goes. I'll need to talk. I don't know what to do. I'm pretty sure Phil wants me to stick to my plans, and I kind of know he's right. But it seems a hard thing to do. I just feel . . . bloody tired, tired of it all, tired of hassle, tired of dreaming and then it all gets fucked up. Perhaps I'd have been better off not dreaming.'

'It may feel that way just now, Mark, but those dreams are real and within your reach. It's just that – and this is going to sound awful, Mark – but the reality is that, well, for whatever reason . . .'

'. . . yeah, I know, my mum doesn't want me to have that dream.'

'Yeah.'

'She needs help, Helen.'

'And she's in the right place. And they need to be aware that she has nowhere to go at the moment where she'll be looked after. They need to keep her in and not let her out too quickly. If they think you'll be there to look after her, well, you'll just get dragged into it all.'

'Yeah. I know. I know.' He sighed heavily.

'Anyway, don't make hasty decisions, Mark, and, yeah, drop over later.'

'I'll see how I'm feeling and what's happening.'

'Anything else you want from us at the moment?'

'No. Thanks for being there, for being around. It helps. I've got some thinking to do and I need to have people around me with sensible heads on. Breakfast's arriving so I may catch up with you later.'

'Sure. And if you want, I can come over later.'

'Yeah, OK. I'll see how it goes.'

'OK. Bye then. Call me if you want me to come over.'

'OK, thanks.'

'Bye. Take care, Mark.'

'Yeah.'

He passed the phone back to Phil. 'I'll be with him for a while, Helen, we'll see how it goes. If anyone phones about needle collection, tell them I'll get back to them, and if they need clean works delivered, well, let Sandy know.' He knew he was a bit out of role, but, well, they didn't have a community support worker, and he was OK with doing this. If it helped someone avoid relapsing it was worth it.

Mark was busy tackling the breakfast. 'Not hungry, huh?'

'Yeah, well.'

They ate in silence. After they'd finished and Phil had paid, they headed back to the ward.

Phil stayed till lunch time. Mark stayed on until early afternoon but then decided that there wasn't anything he could do, and he didn't feel comfortable staying at the hospital. So he took himself back home to Nick and Paula's. He couldn't settle, and decided to head over to the clinic.

At the day programme Judy was passing the card around that she'd bought. After they signed the card the issue was still in the air for the afternoon. A number of people said they were feeling wobbly, feeling really affected by it. More emotion was released. People talked about what support they needed. Some were going to use a little more, no-one said it for definite, but it was in the air. Carrie and Brian sought to encourage them to think of ways of dealing with their feelings, reminding them of the steps they had explored in the previous days. It brought home to both Brian and Carrie just how affected people could be, particularly their clients. Yes, some might see it as a justifiable excuse to use, or use more, but for the most part it was simply people struggling to find ways of dealing with difficult feelings.

Mark changed his mind; he'd go over to the day programme. He kind of felt that somehow that was where he belonged. The feeling had come over him. He could see Helen tomorrow, but somehow, yeah, he just felt he needed to be with the group. He arrived during the mid-afternoon tea break.

They were glad to see him. Judy gave him the card. He read it, felt tears welling up, went to give her a kiss and ended up giving her a big hug and sobbing like a baby on her shoulder. Everyone stood around feeling a mixture of awkwardness and sadness, while also being pleased to see him. One or two reached over and patted him on the back. Mark slowly pulled away and blew out a breath. 'Phew, sorry about that.'

'No need to be sorry, be as you need to be. Really good to see you.' It was another of the participants, Doug. 'I feel I need to give you a hug too.' They embraced, tightly.

'Thanks, Doug. I knew I needed to be here. I'd gone home, then decided to go to the clinic, but then decided that this was where I needed to be. Sorry if I've disrupted things.'

'You've given us so much to work with, today, and sharpened up reality for us.' It was Judy who was speaking. 'Really glad you came over.'

'Do you want to come into the final session, Mark?' Carrie hoped he would; clearly the group was important to him. His being here took some of the not knowing out of everyone's minds and might help those who were feeling wobbly over what had happened.

'Yeah, I'd like that. Just couldn't think of anywhere more important to be.' They were walking into the group room. It was Mark that spoke first once everyone was seated.

'Gonna miss you all next week.' He looked around the circle. He could feel the emotions rising again. Yeah, these people really cared. He thought about the card; he was still holding it. He'd never had a card signed by a whole bunch of people. 'This means so much to me.' He held up the card, and burst into tears again. 'I've never really felt part of a family, but I do here.' He took a deep breath and reined his emotions back in.

'Yeah, me too.'

'And me.'

Everyone was nodding their heads.

It was Doug who asked the question that was on everyone's lips. 'You still going down to Devon, Mark?'

He lifted his hands, then dropped them back on to his thighs. 'You tell me. I don't know.'

'I think you should. You've come so far. You deserve a fresh start, you've worked for it, you've earned it. You're the only one of us that's decided to stop using on this programme, and done it. The rest of still use, or think about using, some more than others I know. You go for it.'

'Thanks, maybe, I don't know. Hard to walk away, you know?'

'I think you need to go as well.' It was Judy this time. 'I mean, I know you need to make up your own mind, and maybe you need to get away to think about it, you know, like I'm doing at the moment. Being with my sister is giving me time to think about what I want, and being here, and I know I'm not going back to my boyfriend now. He's going nowhere and I want to go somewhere. Don't go backwards, Mark, go for it, you deserve it.' She smiled at him, feeling her own emotions rising and the tears oozing over her eyelids. She blinked. 'Shit, you've got me going now as well.'

The group lapsed into silence. But it wasn't awkward, rather a comfortable silence. It was like the silence that happens when everyone knows there is nothing more to say, and no need to say anything about anything else.

Mark took a deep breath. 'Think I need a show of hands. What do you think?'

'Who thinks Mark should go?' It was Doug again. He put his hand up. So did everyone else, even Carrie and Brian.

'I don't have a choice, do I?'

'You always have a choice, Mark.' It was Carrie. 'It's up to you. You've a few more days to decide, and, well, I guess deep down you know what's right for you.'

'Yeah. I do. I have to move on, but I need my mum to understand. I need to try and communicate that somehow, that I'm not abandoning her, but abandoning a way of life. You're right, Judy, I need space and I won't get that round here. Space to think, to make decisions. My mum's being looked after. She's a tough old bird. She'll get through. Maybe if she sees me getting my shit together, maybe things'll change between us. But I can't do it for that, I've got to do it for me.'

'It's the best reason.' Brian was nodding as he spoke.

The group session continued with Mark becoming more sure of his need to stick to his plans. After the session Judy came over. 'Fancy a coffee somewhere?'

'Yeah, thanks, that'll be nice.'

They headed off and sat chatting for a couple of hours. Mark used her mobile to phone the hospital. They said his mum was stable, that they were feeling more positive but she was still drifting in and out of consciousness. They didn't think there was any immediate risk. He said he'd drop in during evening visiting.

They left the café and were heading in different directions. Judy wrote her phone number on a piece of paper and gave it to Mark. 'Call me if you need to talk, any time, and I mean any time.'

'Thanks, Judy.' He gave her a hug. He took a deep breath. It felt good.

'Want me to come to the hospital?'

'That'd be nice, would you? But it must be taking you out of your way.'

'It's OK, it's a nice evening. Nothing to rush back for. I can call my sister, say I'll be back later.'

They headed off to the hospital together.

Tuesday 12 September – care co-ordination

'So, you're really in two minds about what to do?'

Mark nodded. He'd really enjoyed being with Judy the previous evening. They'd really hit it off. The thought of heading away now seemed even harder. But he also knew that he had to. But it left him feeling very mixed up.

'I know I have to – the group's right, I have to give myself a chance, give myself space, take the opportunity that's there for me.'

Helen really felt for him. Her own view was that he needed to move away, get himself together and then, well, he could make other decisions at some later time. But she also appreciated that this was drugs work. Things changed fast and the need for adaptability was enormous.

'I guess my perspective, as your care co-ordinator, is that I need to be thinking through what can be most helpful for you should you decide to stay. I mean, we need to cover all the angles, so to speak.'

'I'm sure I'm not staying. Even if the worst happens – she dies – and that seems less likely now, well, I'd still feel I needed a fresh start, you know?'

'Yeah. OK. So we continue to work towards you heading off at the weekend to start your new life.' Helen wanted to keep it positive. 'And the group ends on Thursday, and you've ended with Tony, and we see you for the last time on Friday.'

Mark took a deep breath. 'Yeah. Talk about everything happening at once.'

Nature's way, thought Helen, but she kept her thought to herself. She simply said, 'Sometimes that seems how it goes.'

They took time to discuss Mark's particular anxieties. Most of it was about leaving his mother, or at least, how would he tell her, would she understand? The hospital was happy that she was pulling through. He knew he should spend more time with her, and he was heading off after the session with Helen. He hoped to then meet Judy later as well.

'What do I say to her? I mean, she's got to know.'

'Yeah, I think you owe that to each other.'

Mark was shaking his head. 'I mean, I'm still angry with her, and I'm also not surprised. Should have been prepared for it.'

'Could you have made any difference though?'

'No. But it's really tough knowing what to say.'

'What do you want to say?'

'I have to go. This is for me. I've got to change, else I'll just ...' He shrugged. 'Risk is I'll slide back on to the gear again. Too many people round here. Too much opportunity.'

'I think you've got to go with what you believe to be right for you.'

'Thanks for all the support and everything; you've really made it happen.'

'Hey, I'm glad to have been of help, to make a difference. They sound a really positive and innovative team where you're going. I feel good about what I've read and heard about them.'

Mark was suddenly feeling very drained and emotional. 'I'm going to miss this. Without this place and the people here, well, I might not be here. Still got a lot to face up to though, a lot to sort out in my head.'

'Yeah, and you will. You'll get the help you need to do it, and then, well, fresh opportunities.'

'I said I want to get into this kind of work. Rod's looked out some basic counselling courses – I'm going to enrol and get a feel for it.'

'Sounds good. Find something that feels right for you, Mark. But also be aware of not getting too close to the drug world while it's still too close to you.'

'I like that, yeah, sums it up, yeah, that's good.' He smiled.

They continued the session, Helen checking that he had the contact details for the service in Devon. He confirmed that he had.

'What about Phil, seeing him again this week?'

'Seeing him later today, meeting up after I've been to the hospital. And maybe see him at the end of the week, I don't know, I'll have a lot of sorting out to do, and a few more goodbyes to people.'

'OK. Well, I'm glad we drafted him in.'

'Me too. It was good to see him yesterday. Just having someone around, and the breakfast was good too!' He smiled as he looked Helen in the eye.

'Yes, I heard about that – not hungry!'

'Yeah, well, you know.'

The session ended and Mark made his way to the hospital. His mother was sitting up in bed. She smiled as he came in.

'Been thinking about you, thinking about a lot of things. I'm still fuzzy but I do feel a bit more together.'

'Yeah.' Mark could feel the anxiety as his heart thudded in his chest. He knew he had to tell her but, oh God, it wasn't going to be easy. 'Look, mum, I know this is tough for you and everything but ...'

'... you're still going, aren't you?'

He nodded, and he suddenly felt quite tearful. His eyes were watering.

His mum had noticed it, and she was touched by it; first time he'd shown emotion like that towards her for the longest while.

'I know I don't want you to go, but I know what I did was stupid. I just lost it.'

'I know. It's OK. But I'll come back and visit. Look, I'm clean now, been drug-free since last week, well, the end of. And in spite of all this, I'm going to stay that way. Been getting a lot of help, a lot of support. And I want to stay this way. I need to be in another space to do that, but I'll come back to visit, and maybe you could come down to me, Rod's said that'll be OK.'

They continued in conversation. Something had changed between them. Neither could quite define what it was, but somehow it seemed for Mark that he had got his mum back, and she had got a son again. Neither spoke of this, but there was a closeness between them that hadn't existed in years.

The door opened and Phil came in. Mark introduced him to his mum, and they headed off. He promised to drop back later, which he did, leaving Judy waiting for him which she was happy to do.

Thursday 14 September – day programme
The final day was spent processing endings, and to begin with Mark was quite withdrawn. He was so full of endings; he felt he needed to take his time. They had a quiz about drugs to help people realise what they had learned. They looked at people's hopes for the future, what they were taking away with them, what their next steps were. Throughout the day Mark and Judy were smiling at each other, finding time during the coffee and tea breaks to chat. In the afternoon session Mark spoke at length, about his own process and of the hopes he had for his new life. They then began expressing feelings towards each other, going through an exercise offering each other positive qualities that they saw in each other. And suddenly it was time to leave.

No-one seemed in a rush to leave; everyone felt good and was finding it hard to go. But eventually they did. Mark left with Judy; they headed out to the hospital and then later back to her sister's for a meal. Mark set off back to Nick and Paula's feeling so many things. It felt strange. But it felt good. It sort of felt like there was stuff going on inside him and his head had a lot of catching up to do to make sense of it all.

Friday 15 September – clinic and care co-ordination
Dr Ashton was very positive and encouraging, saying how pleased he was with his progress and how he wished him all the best. He checked that he hadn't had any adverse reactions to finally stopping the buprenorphine. He said no, although with everything that had been happening it was hard to know where his feelings were coming from. Dr Ashton explained that he had written to the team in Devon, and explained what he had said. He'd been very positive though he had also mentioned some of the difficulties that had occurred over recent weeks. They shook hands and Mark went into the other room with Helen.

'So, you're off.'

Mark nodded.

'Anything further you need from us?'

Mark shook his head.

'Before you go I need you to complete a short questionnaire for our records.'

'That's OK.'

Completing it involved him defining his level of confidence, how positive he felt, what his mood was like, and some more practical things like drug use – nil. He smiled at that one, though he did have to admit that, yes, he was drinking a bit most days.

'Think I've said enough about that in the past. Please keep an eye on it, Mark.'

'I know.'

So the session came to an end and Mark headed off, after giving Helen a hug. It felt a really natural thing to do, somehow. He really was grateful for all the help and now, well, now was the future, a new start. Rod was coming the next day and they were going to visit his mother before they left. He wanted to see her, reassure her. And then . . . He was full of his own thoughts as he strolled down the corridor, and almost walked into Judy who was waiting for him. They left, arm in arm, maybe another new beginning. Only time would tell.

Summary

Mark's mother overdoses; he calls the day programme who liaise with Mark's care co-ordinator. The outreach worker goes to the hospital to be with Mark and to try to offer him support through it. Mark is unclear what to do, whether to continue with his plans, or stay. Mark goes to the day programme in the afternoon and they vote on it. He also spends time with Judy from the programme; they get on really well. He talks to Helen and realises he has to move away. He talks to his mother – it is an emotional conversation. He has decided to leave.

PART 3

Reflecting on the success of Models of Care for this patient

CHAPTER 10

Reflections

From overdose to a new start in life. Mark's story may seem compressed. Often the journey is longer, but sometimes it can happen more quickly, depending on circumstances, the client's readiness to change, and the support and treatment responses that are made available. Many people were involved in Mark's journey. The following professionals each played their part.

Tony

'I thought Mark did well. He came through a lot of shit to get his opportunity. Some of the sessions were hard going, so much anger, and then the sadness for his loss. He could have blown it; he did stupid things and he knew it. He could have lost his script perhaps, or not re-engaged with the service. But something kept him trying.

'It always fills me with a sense of achievement when I see someone changing in such a way that they are more authentically present. Mark came in still under the influence of methadone and with a lot of drug-related thinking in his head. He took a brave decision to seek clarity and to face his feelings. I admire him for that. Not everyone is prepared to do this, preferring the drug-induced numbness to the sharp pain of reality. I heard later about his mother's overdose, when I got back from holiday. My heart went out to Mark. Was he OK? What had happened? Had he stuck to his resolve? Yes he had, and I was grateful. And I thought about his mum, another tragic victim of drug use, left with anxieties that at times were unmanageable. But maybe now there might be some healing for her through the changes in Mark. I hope so.'

Dr Ashton

'Clinical responsibility weighs heavily sometimes when clients are chaotic in their drug use. Mark was not the worst, by any means. But he did push things. We gave him what we felt he needed medically. We took a risk. We could have said, no more, after he'd used on top of the methadone, when he used again this time on top of the buprenorphine, but then what? He'd have used more no doubt, and put himself at greater risk. Yes, it was risky prescribing – he was still drinking too – but what was the alternative? It seemed there was an opportunity for Mark if we could get him through it, and particularly with the support that was available, and the different treatments that he was engaging with. He was clearly motivated, but struggling at times.

'He did remarkably well, and yet in many ways the process has barely begun. Letting go of the old ways, the old patterns of dealing with things is one thing; creating something new is a different process. But he has the opportunity now. I hope he makes it. He may not. Things happen in the world of drug use, and happen fast. Some feeling might overwhelm him and in a moment of temptation he slips up. But let's hope not. I'm glad to have played a part in his recovery.'

Carrie and Brian

'He really used the group well, and I think got so much from it. He really did seem motivated and was really prepared to be open and share his experience. The issue with Mandy seemed a turning point, somehow. He wasn't prepared to hide behind anything. He knew he'd done something stupid and felt safe enough to own it. I know that actually made a big impact on the group.

'When the group voted for him to go the atmosphere was electric. Neither of us had experienced anything quite like that before, and we were swept along by it. We had our hands up as well. We just knew he had to move on.

'We had been a little hesitant over the medication switch and the detoxification, but then, what was the alternative? He waits for the next programme? No, it just felt like Mark was making choices for himself and it felt appropriate to fit services around that. It could otherwise get far too "treatment-centred". Mark knew what he wanted to go for and it felt right to give him a chance, give him the support and be prepared to help him if things got really difficult. It felt very "client-centred" in the widest sense of the term.'

Phil

'Mark? I liked him. Poor guy. He had some stuff to wade through, but he changed. He wasn't the person that last week that I met when he was in hospital. Just wanted to use then, no thoughts of stopping. And yet, he changed, he moved – literally – and it was good to have worked with him. I was a bit out of role that last week, but he needed time with someone and I could offer that. And then there was Judy; she helped that last week. He talked a lot about her.

'I like to think that my first contact with him in the hospital encouraged him to come in to the clinic. Maybe something I'd said, the way I was. I'm glad he did come in. Never could get him on his mobile. No, he made the decision to seek help, and I'm sure that came out of that first informal contact with him. So, a good job done. That's what outreach is all about – making contact, getting the harm minimisation message across, and drawing people into treatment services.'

Helen

'Something about him, right from the start. I think he pulled on some mothering urge in me, as I look back on it all now. And, yes, I got fired up with him once or twice. Perhaps as much my own frustration as anything else. I was carrying a high caseload and there just never seemed enough processing time. That's changing now. It's such intense work, care co-ordination. You have to be so aware of what's happening, trying to be a step ahead all of the time. I guess that's the difference between me and Tony. He stays by their side; I have to be a step ahead a lot of the time. But that's OK; it works well.

'He made it to Devon, but, shit, it was close. That's drug work. Don't believe anything will happen till it happens. Things do happen fast. One moment all seems plain sailing and then ... Bit like walking in the snow and then you step on an icy slope and you're falling. It could all have been so different at so many stages. But he stuck at it and we stuck with him. In a way I suppose we all took risks. But that's it, isn't it? Drugs are about risk. People are either dealing with the emotional and psychological fall-out from being in risky environments, or seeking to perpetuate feelings associated with risk, or the risk is just the simple effect of injecting whatever the dealer decides to cut with your drug. And the psychological effect of the drug itself. More and more drugs – designer drugs, more concentrated drugs – what the long-term effects will be only time will tell. It's risk all the way. We try to minimise it, but can you ever completely cut it out?

'I enjoy care co-ordination though it is stressful. It's good to feel able to pull things together and to work with other staff and agencies collaboratively. It's a bit of a buzz really, seeing it all come together.

'But what would have happened if Mark had lost his script for using on top? What would have happened if he'd broken contact when he'd been using? What would have happened if he hadn't broken away from Mandy? What would have happened if he had stayed behind with his mum and they had resolved nothing between them? Nothing's ever simple working in this speciality; nothing can be taken for granted. It's not easy breaking a habit, particularly when the habit involves the use of powerful and dependence-forming chemicals.'

Mark

'It's great here, time on the beach, time to make new friends. Got into surfing. Started chatting to a couple of guys down here one night and, well, I'm really into it now. I'm working for my cousin, and that's going well. Got settled into that. Bloody hard work, and my muscles were really aching when I started. But figured it'd be good for me, build myself up. And I feel good about it now, feel good in myself.

'I'm still with the local drug and alcohol team. Seeing a counsellor, been going there for six months now. Still wading through stuff from the past and making sense of decisions I'm taking in the present.

'Somehow the past seems kind of unreal and yet all too real as well. I'm in a different world here. Not just the environment; it's what's in my head. I have only been back a couple of times; I don't like it, too many memories. Mum has come down here twice. First time we had to go and collect her; the second time she took the train. Anxious as ever, but she made it. Things are a little easier. How easy it will get, time will tell.

'And Judy? Well, we see each other, you know, she's still at her sister's but isn't going back to her boyfriend – talking about coming down here. That's one of the things I talk about a lot in the counselling. I like her a lot, but do I like her enough? Relationships. I don't really understand them – more of the fall-out from the past.

'So, I feel really grateful and still coming to terms with it all. But I have a life and I'm enjoying it. Still have a few beers, but I know I'm drinking for a different reason now. It's social. I'm not trying to get away from stuff. Something in me has moved on; it's just that old ways of thinking and feeling about things come back at me now and then. And I know how different it could have been. I still remember the "no change" life line – how much shorter it was. More than anything else, that somehow made an impression on me – and Helen getting fired up about my drinking and everything. Yeah, I'm learning to accept that people care about me, and that I deserve to be cared about. And I'm also learning to care about myself, too. Anything goes won't do any more. And that's quite a lot to adjust to as well.'

Reflecting on Mark's journey through Models of Care: a psychiatrist's perspective*

A journey that needs a clear road map

Mark is embarking on a journey that must be mapped out from the start if Models of Care is to have any meaning and not present the patient, as user, with another nostrum for the new century. The stages must be negotiable and easily understood, both by Mark and similar clients, and by the array of professionals involved in its implementation. The concept is noble and vast. There are large numbers of professionals involved, working at different levels, in a variety of organisations. All are hoping for the best outcome for the patient, whatever that might be.

Models of Care is not easy ...

As Edward de Bono remarked, the difference between our talents and expectations is disappointment. We are trying not to disappoint our clients while empowering our staff. We are looking for the best of care. This will ride on a template that attempts to ensure easy access to treatment, quality at all levels and a management plan. This latter must be understandable to all who access it, irrespective of the timeframe, from within the multidisciplinary teams involved but also by those pursuing similar documented care plans that have been replicated nationwide.

It may appear as though we are staring into the chasm that exists between the suggesting and the implementation of this tall order. On the other hand, without it, Mark would have been left to the vagaries of the system that existed before. Now there may be a chance for people like him to get help that will lead to recovery.

* This section has been written by **William Shanahan** MB DCH FRCPsych, Lead Clinician, Substance Misuse Service, Central and North West London Mental Health NHS Trust, and Executive Medical Director, Florence Nightingale Hospitals.

In accepting the Models of Care, we may, at the very least, give ourselves a foundation from which to grow even if we do not grow quickly.

Previously, in the drug treatment world, Mark's experience would have been hit and miss. He would have been exposed to the prevailing emotions of the service within which he surfaced. Arbitrary decisions, based on historical precedents arising from the personal experience of individuals, tended to shape the clinical response. This so-called experience was often nothing more than a bevy of erroneous, albeit well-meaning, assumptions set on a time loop. There was no evidence base. Care could be very good or very bad. There was no triage system and, in many centres, substitute prescribing failed to meet the needs of the client. Furthermore, there was little understanding of the problems imposed by a dual diagnosis in this client group.

The Models of Care system hopes to surmount all of these difficulties by defining roles and responsibilities for both the client and the carer. However, the system will be client-centred. At the heart of this lies the hope that the delivery of the care required will be co-ordinated, planned, reviewed, researched and evaluated. The professionals will be trained and supervised. They will undergo appraisal and adhere to the requirements of clinical governance and risk management. They will be familiar with the concept of integrated care pathways and they will know where to go when they run into trouble.

How well does Mark's story match real-life experiences?

In this story, Mark receives a very comprehensive treatment package. The system appears to flow and the model works in a way that will gladden the hearts of the architects of this concept. Is it realistic? I think not, because it presumes that all of the players have bought into the model and have a reasonably clear understanding of their own roles and limitations. It is unlikely to be as simple as this in real life, where the boundaries will be much more blurred, and many of the people involved will want to do more and, sometimes, even less than they are doing here.

Phil's role in assessment

From the start, Phil is self-assured and aware. Some might argue that his rather foul-mouthed approach to the client is a dubious quality. He has the menu off pat – 'substitute prescribing, counselling, relapse prevention, maybe some social work input' – but the assessment is confusing. Is he just the warm-up act or is he meant to be getting some useful background information relevant to an assessment? Problems with role definition surface later in the story as workers try to make sense of their limitations.

Where does the GP fit in?

These difficulties are worth noting, because they are likely to be encountered in the real world, where any confusion about who should be doing what, among the staff, will be reflected in the client group. Does the implementation of this idea preclude the notion that, sometimes and somewhere, one professional may be more important or more significant in the life of the client than another? We learn, well into the book, that Mark has a GP. He or she may have known Mark since birth and may also know his difficult mother.

Ignoring such a valuable source of information, especially early on in the assessment process, risks throwing the baby out with the bath water. If Models of Care tries to homogenise the relevance of the professionals involved with the client, we increase the likelihood of losing everything that was useful about the old form of assessment. Where does the doctor fit in? Indeed, the role of the medical staff is difficult to define in this scenario.

Other care professionals

This happy place also has a group of nurses, therapeutic counsellors, day hospital workers and local authority employees, all of whom are ready and willing to don their respective mantles and take their places on the treatment stage, under the careful direction of the treatment co-ordinator. Really, how long will it be before we can hope for anything approaching this utopia? A world where telephones get answered, post arrives on time and everyone gets along just fine seems such a nice idea.

What happens to Mark if some of the clinical staff disagree about planning or change their minds? What if there are personal problems between people in different services? The usual capacity problems can, in themselves, disrupt the care planning and lead to a disenchanted client dropping out of treatment. At present, 50% of clients leave treatment early. Will the Models of Care really address this without a serious overhaul of existing services and an appreciation of the funding that will be required for this?

But Models of Care is succeeding

On the positive side, some services, including special Tier 4A clinics, are already satisfying many of the aspirations laid out in the Models of Care documentation. There is a sense of increasing access to services in several boroughs. Robust tolerance testing assures the clients of adequate doses of medication and a comfortable stabilisation period. There is security of tenure within the clinic and clients are not discharged for doing well just because a certain time period has elapsed.

But there are potential pitfalls ahead

There are inherent contradictions in this that must be recognised. The successful operation of Models of Care depends on client throughput and availability of treatment slots. At the same time the clients who manage to access treatment are being promised lengthy periods of substitute prescribing while being encouraged to consider abstinence at some point. This will inevitably lead to capacity problems and blockages in the system. Client advocates will then complain of poor access to initial assessment and care managers will find it impossible to move clients from one service to another and therefore from one tier to another.

Who leads the team: the changing role of the consultant

Mark's story offers a clear demonstration of the challenges facing various professionals involved in the care of people like him. What it also does is shift the emphasis from consultant-led teams that make all the decisions, to a more holistic form of care management in which workers and teams respond to a client's needs as they arise, under the watchful eye of a care co-ordinator. This raises questions in itself. Who is actually in charge? Are we entering a phase of democratic management?

Mark's problems are not discussed at a multidisciplinary team meeting. The presumption is that one doctor will prescribe much like another. This is a long way from being the case. Some consultants are likely to react very badly to the loss of a clearly defined team leadership role. There is a feeling already that this version of the National Service Framework has been introduced too rapidly and without proper consultation with the medical people who previously managed the Drug Treatment Clinics and signed all the prescriptions.

Historically, consultants have been psychiatrists. The behavioural problems accompanying substance misuse, along with the alteration in mental state, has dictated this. In this story, the doctors could as easily be community health physicians or specialist GPs. Where this will matter most will be in the emerging problems with dual diagnoses. How will Models of Care tie in the large numbers of young people currently using 'skunk' and other forms of cannabis? Will Adult Mental Health Services accept the opinion of the co-ordinator that a more comprehensive CPA is required for a psychotic user? Will the inpatient unit?

Models of Care: challenges ahead

This book sets out one man's journey through stages of treatment with care and illustrates how it might work. At its core, and at the centre of the whole package, is the presumption that the client is at least partially motivated to enter the system. The staff are nice and friendly and the clinics have space. The idea is a good one and deserves a chance. The challenges will be many and will be delivered by many routes: the physically ill patient with multiple disabilities and the DTTO (Drug Treatment and Testing Orders) person and other police referrals. The problems with follow-up, aftercare, governance and disgruntled staff will be some of the hurdles.

Finally, there are the prescribing problems. How client-led can this be? What happens when one service refuses to continue a drug regime commenced in another? Clearly, time and training will be required for all players. More treatment, fairer treatment, better treatment, and the money to help deliver it all, may get Mark and similar people the care they need and deserve.

Reflecting on Mark's journey through Models of Care: a family therapy perspective*

Reading Mark's story one could easily be forgiven for thinking of him not so much as a member of a family but as an individual who has to overcome formidable obstacles, not least of which is his mother's planned overdose.

The family therapist is tuned into *change* that is taking place at several different levels among those affected by the user's – Mark's – decision to confront his drug use. The family therapist takes into consideration the dynamic interaction within family relationships and formulates a working hypothesis to help make sense of the possible pitfalls that could undermine a carefully organised treatment plan.

Mark's story is a good case in point. We're introduced to Mark's family history quite early on. He has only to think of altering his relationship to drug taking when disturbing thoughts and emotions relating to his mother, and problems associated with family history, come bubbling to the surface. Knowledge of these family dynamics can play a significant role in helping clients like Mark to recognise that those 'significant others' are, and will be, affected by the change he's planning to make. The family therapist brings a point of view that looks at the bigger picture, taking into consideration the various perspectives and potential conflicts held by other members of the family. Family patterns of interaction are just that, patterns, and as such are predictable and useful in assessing how the family discusses problems, change and solutions. When members of a family are faced with one of their own choosing to alter their way of life in some crucial way, their behaviour could be construed as a way of preserving the status quo. Though this is not at all outside the norm, in Mark's case several professionals, closely involved in monitoring his progress, fell prey to the notion that his mother's overdose was an act of 'sabotage', rather than a misguided attempt at keeping the family together.

Neither should it be assumed that in a different context – one where Mark's mother is invited to consider her best hopes for her son's 'noble intention' to become drug-free – she wouldn't respond with her full support. The family therapist

---

* This section has been written by the Substance Misuse Family Therapy Service, Central and North West London Mental Health NHS Trust.

brings a professional skill which helps the family overcome the behaviours and beliefs that make change unsettling. A way of achieving this with Mark's mother would be for the therapist to shift attention away from Mark towards his mother in order to discuss how his planned change in drug use could 'positively' affect her life and improve her relationship with her son.

This example is but one of several possible interventions for a specialist structured family therapy interview. Such an intervention could have occurred around the time Mark had achieved drug-free status and when plans were moving swiftly ahead to transfer himself and his treatment to Devon. With hindsight we can almost hear his mother waving her arms in the background saying, 'What about me?'

A Tier 3 referral may have helped smooth the way for a less disturbing transition but the question should also be asked, how might Mark's care co-ordinator have taken these issues into consideration sooner? As care co-ordinator, Helen had to organise a plan that helped Mark to move cautiously and carefully through the early stages of his treatment. The issues being grappled with were many, and though they were all connected in some way to Mark's decision to 'do something', at this delicate time Mark first needed to find that he could trust other people to help him. Until Mark had formulated in his own mind *what* he wanted from his treatment, a referral to the specialist family therapist may well have proven counterproductive. Care co-ordinators, like Helen, may serve their clients better by exploring more fully how the client's nearest and dearest are likely to be affected by their decision to address their use of drugs. Having a leaflet with information designed to be given to the relative by the client is another way of acknowledging that the client is aware of those others and their need for help. Such information should include advice on support groups as well as other options for those members of the family who may wish to use help for themselves. In Mark's day programme, psycho-education sessions could be planned to help illustrate how those family dynamics discussed above may play out. The role of family therapy can facilitate a transition to a future where the family members and their dynamic interplay can make a choice to adjust differently to a new life style.

Reviewing the clinical literature

Meta-studies within the drug and alcohol field, e.g. Stanton and Standish (1997) and Edwards and Steinglass (1995) and O'Farrell (1995) respectively, suggest family therapy is a useful adjunct to medical approaches and is seen as a more beneficial form of psychotherapy than individual or group approaches.

Within the family therapy paradigm the therapist has many different approaches that might help Mark consider his changing relationships to both his drug use and his mother. Using these approaches means adopting a post-structural stance in that the therapist would work collaboratively with the client towards their desired goals.

Milan approaches (Boscolo *et al.*, 1987) would look at Mark's (and his mother's) beliefs, perhaps about family functioning or drug use, and include different perspectives from significant others (family members, different workers involved in his care, etc.) and over time. In this way past changes, future choices and the impact of these on his family and other parts of his system can be explored.

A trans-generational framework (Byng-Hall, 1995) would explore patterns (scripts) of family dynamics and drug difficulties, how these were handled over different generations, e.g. the impact of his mother's use, and the impact of these on Mark's dilemmas. Looking at ways these scripts could be replicated or corrected in their present situation might be useful for Mark and his mother.

Narrative approaches (White, 1989) would look carefully at the language used to describe his difficulties. By deconstructing these descriptions Mark might find that difficulties in making changes to his life were amplified by *embedded expectations* (dominant narratives themes) of others, e.g. attitudes of family, drug agencies or society. Objectifying these difficulties and re-authoring and witnessing more useful, subjugated narratives that see Mark moving in a direction he wants might liberate him to make changes that are useful to him.

A solution-focused approach (DeShazer, 1991) could look at goals and what their preferred future would look like (maybe in terms of Mark seeing himself drug-free or having a good relationship with his mother). Subsequently, the therapist helps explore what progress they have made towards this and what it would look like if things further moved in the right direction.

References

- Boscolo L, Cecchin G, Hoffman L and Penn P (1987) *Milan Systemic Family Therapy: conversations in theory and practice*. Basic Books, New York.

- Byng-Hall J (1995) *Re-writing Family Scripts*. Guilford Press, New York.

- DeShazer S (1991) *Putting Difference to Work*. Norton, New York.

- Edwards M and Steinglass P (1995) Family therapy treatment outcomes for alcoholics. *Journal of Marital and Family Therapy*. **21**(4): 475–509.

- O'Farrell T (1995) Marital and family therapy. In: R Hester and W Miller (eds) *Handbook of Alcoholism Treatment Approaches*. Allyn and Bacon, New York.

- Stanton MD and Standish WR (1997) Outcome, attrition and family-couples treatment for drug abuse. *Psychological Bulletin*. **122**(2): 170–91.

- White M (1989) *Selected Papers*. Dulwich Centre Publications, Adelaide.

Emerging themes: reflections of a nurse consultant*

The initial contact is vital for engaging service users. Life-threatening events may actually force service users to contemplate decisions that will change patterns of behaviour. It is important not to underestimate the impact of how health and social care professionals relate to clients. Over-familiarity in approach is not necessarily helpful from some professionals and could be perceived as disrespectful by the service user, e.g. using the term 'mate'. For Phil, working as a frontline outreach worker, it seems that he had devised an approach that seemed to work for him. However, this approach may not be appropriate for everyone. Phil attempts to engage Mark by addressing the options that are available to him as he recovers from an overdose. Authenticity within the relationship and the use of language are important factors when engaging service users – trying to be on the 'same level' or perceived as knowing what a service user is experiencing, may actually be disrespectful.

Managing risk and risk behaviour are key when working with service users, as the very nature of substance misuse may involve high-risk behaviours such as injecting illicit drugs and possibly sharing equipment. This can be managed at different times through a variety of strategies and interventions. An example of immediate risk management is explained by Phil when teaching Mark about the risks of drug overdose. Mark's friends intervened to save his life by recognising the danger signs of overdose. In many ways this may appear to be a contradiction – on the one hand services are provided to address the levels of substance misuse, and on the other there's the reality that a harm minimisation approach is required. Substance misuse is increasing in prevalence so health education for the population is essential to minimise health risks.

Discussion of the pharmacological effects of drugs and alcohol and the impact of drugs on the body with self-medication occurs frequently. Service users may use substances (drugs and/or alcohol) to deal with their psychological distress, as illustrated by Mark's use of alcohol and benzodiazepines. Poly-drug use may

* This section has been written by **Caroline Frayne**, Nurse Consultant, Substance Misuse Service, Central and North West London Mental Health NHS Trust.

be reflective of using chemicals to resolve emotional difficulties of stress and anxiety. Treatment encompasses many modalities from pharmacology to psychological interventions. Helen highlights the importance of using interventions that focus on helping Mark address his personal difficulties. This also entails supporting Mark to understand how medication can impact on his treatment outcomes. Dr Ashton prescribes methadone (which is the substitute choice of treatment for heroin dependency) as part of the treatment plan. The section detailing aspects of Mark's monitoring also addresses the purpose of urine toxicology as a treatment intervention. This not only ensures Mark is taking the medication prescribed by Dr Ashton, but also engages him in monitoring his progress. What is considered a core intervention can also be a source of contention as continued treatment is partly dependent upon the results.

Multi-professional liaison and communication are key responsibilities for Helen as the nominated care co-ordinator, and this requires liaison with a variety of health and social care professionals. Helen lets Mark know that she will inform the GP of his treatment. Even though Mark will be attending the treatment team for supervised consumption of methadone, he may still need to visit his GP for any general medical service. To ensure successful co-ordination of Mark's care, Helen must establish a therapeutic relationship which requires negotiation of Mark's health information and protection and prevention through all services. It is important to manage misinformation about services. When contemplating assessment any Tier 3 service should include health, physical, psychological and social assessment. Helen uses the Life Line tool to assist Mark in making decisions. The main focus is on assisting clients to manage their drug use so they can develop skills and strategies to manage their feelings and family relationships. Referral to the Day Programme, and its structured groups, provides the environment in which to explore difficulties.

Helen identifies the importance of awareness of the boundaries of her own role in supporting Mark. Helen acknowledges Jim's role in providing a humanistic counselling environment in which Mark can explore his difficulties. She monitors Mark's progress and she is the central communication point for all the professionals providing care for Mark. In her role as overseer Helen may be required to raise difficult issues with clients, she will need to manage any concerns that a professional may have and be aware of the service user's agenda. Some first-time service users may take a different view of risk and be unable to see the broader picture – therefore there can be conflict over the main priorities. Staff also have to manage their own anxieties about the service user's management of drug and/or alcohol use. Working with service users who have emotional problems can be draining for staff, and supervision is essential to allow staff to reflect on their work with clients. Professional network forums are an effective and useful way of addressing communication and liaison issues. Given Mark's history of overdosing, the professional network's concern for his well-being is understandable.

There are difficulties for staff when dealing with personal disclosure – the question is, how much disclosure? Perhaps the question should be, why any disclosure at all? How will it benefit the client, if at all? No two service users present with the same problems or difficulties, and they can be reluctant to seek help from service providers who will disclose personal information.

There is a strong need for developing trust between the professional and the service user. We know that using drugs involves an element of risk behaviour and that establishing relationships with clients can be risky, as they may not engage. Working with clients to address their difficulties and developing trusting relationships involve an element of risk. Service users have to decide the pros and cons of disclosing difficulties, as not only could this impact on their relationship with their workers, but also on the chance of losing treatment.

For all the agencies working with Mark, the importance of clear protocols about sharing information and confidentiality is highlighted. When a client's decision may not match the professional's advice, the service must manage their own anxieties and perceptions. Mark's perception of his alcohol use was that it was not a problem. However, Helen was right to address this issue with Mark as there is clear evidence of the relationship between drug interactions and alcohol and drug use.

From both personal and professional perspectives, working with substance misuse is challenging, causing one to reflect at length on whether we are providing an appropriate service that meets the needs of a vulnerable client group. However, it is important to remain positive and to believe that, given appropriate services and support, service users can make positive changes. This book highlights the importance of communication and the way in which services and professionals can come together to offer the opportunity for change in clients who are pursuing a risky lifestyle and who initially present with no thoughts of change.

Conclusion

I am very grateful to Dr Shanahan for contributing his experienced view of the treatment Mark receives, and the areas where there is highlighted the potential for lack of role clarity and problems in efficient service delivery. He ably raises areas of concern that need to be taken into account in the implementation process. Yes, the story is in a sense idealistic – how it could work – and, yes, the real-world experience will, no doubt, at times be different, as Dr Shanahan points out. Services must be mindful of this, ensuring clarity of professional roles and responsibilities, clear liaison links and a wholehearted willingness to embrace a collaborative approach.

Caroline Frayne has also offered a valuable perspective, giving a nursing view of the treatment process and highlighting important areas to be considered. Initial contact – it can establish the basis for a good working relationship or generate a barrier that may never be fully overcome. Risk assessment and management – people using substances are choosing a risky lifestyle. How can this most effectively be managed by service providers and the users themselves, and what is the meaning and role that the client attaches to their choice to take such risks? She also emphasises the need for a multi-disciplinary approach to ensure that clients do receive the treatment they require. Models of Care should encourage a cohesive and collaborative response and the establishing of clear protocols, well-defined treatment modalities and care pathways and open systems of communication between individual professionals and service providers. The complexity that arises from the cocktail of substances that may be being used is highlighted, together with the need for those who work in the substance misuse field to have appropriate levels of supervision, support and on-going professional development. Yes, the client group can be demanding and ways to deal with this need to be formulated and applied for everyone's benefit. But we must not forget, as Caroline also points out, that this is a very vulnerable group of people. I am grateful for her reflection which focuses our thinking on these fundamental themes for working in the substance misuse field.

So, with these thoughts in mind, we see Mark moves on to a new life. And yet there were many times when he might not have reached his goal. Some of these critical moments were self-induced, and they could have been exacerbated by different responses from the drug services involved in his treatment, or the experience of a reduced range of services not working in such a co-operative manner. Resolving problematic drug use is, by its very nature, a problematic process in the sense that it is never a simple process. Established attitudes and patterns of behaviour need to be addressed, and as well as the psychological and emotional processes connected with drug-using behaviour, there will also be that added complication of the chemical effects on the brain that themselves contribute to the urge to use.

Mark moves on to a fresh start in his life in another location; however, he could have remained in the same area given the events towards the end of the story. In such an instance, whether or not he lapses back into substance use, a review of his care plan might have drawn in other professionals and treatment modalities. Had he stayed for his mother, it might have led to a recognised need for some form of family therapy to help them work on their relationship. Often substance misuse is an aspect of a family system that has been, or remains, problematic, with the substance use by an individual (or individuals) seemingly a symptom of the family system. How much might Mark have to work on his relationship to his mother to resolve underlying emotions and drives to use? And would she have to work on her relationship with him to contribute to the effectiveness of his therapeutic process?

I am grateful for the family therapy perspective on the story. Drug use is often taking place within the context of a relational system – the family being a primary one. The role of familial experience in contributing to drug use is a topic in itself and is not the subject of this volume. Yet it is a perspective that drug services should embrace, perhaps more fully. Treatment of a drug user is likely to be more effective when this takes place in the context of therapeutic and educational processes for the other members of the family system.

As Models of Care becomes fully implemented, it will be vital for care co-ordinators to develop a fuller, working appreciation of the contributions that different professionals can make to the process of treatment and care of individual drug users and those affected by their drug-using behaviours. We can see, from Mark's story, how other professionals might have been involved, and may still play a valuable part in aiding and supporting him in his process of recovery.

There might have been a need for psychological intervention to help him to resolve cognitive patterns and behaviours that had become firmly established as part of his substance-using lifestyle. Or perhaps some form of creative expression might have formed part of his rehabilitation process, or encouragement into new forms of social integration, which could have involved occupational therapy services.

Mark may have found himself in debt or with a housing problem, if his friends had chosen not to continue to house him, leaving him in need of social support. He could have found himself in need of social worker input. Had the detoxification not been successful, he may have had to consider an inpatient detoxification and/ or a residential rehabilitation programme. Again, this would have generated the need for another care pathway to be integrated into the care plan.

Getting back to work could also have been an issue. A need for attendance at some form of community support programme to help him gain a sense of commitment to a work routine may have become a necessary factor in his recovery, or one of the schemes established around the country with the remit to help people move from dependency back into the world of employment.

Mark might have not had the opportunity to move out of the area, but rather chosen to remain on a steady methadone prescription, being maintained at a tolerable level of use. Had he stabilised successfully then he might have been referred back to his GP for ongoing care and prescribing – initially with the support of the substance misuse service but perhaps later able to proceed with only his GP's input. The need to develop strong liaison links with primary healthcare services can be a vital component in moving stabilised clients out of the often more intense Tier 3 treatment services, freeing up space for other clients, who are perhaps more chaotic in their use, to be given the opportunity of a stabilisation programme and/or other treatment options.

Mark might have had other problems associated with his injecting drug use: hepatitis or other blood-borne viruses, or HIV, are common. Packages of treatment and care may have needed to have been formulated to respond to these: another care pathway requiring integration into the treatment package.

The truth is that in this fictitious account Mark is, to some degree, fortunate, but he has also been offered the opportunity to ride his luck and establish changes. Not all will reach the point that he has. Death and serious debilitating and damaging health conditions can and do occur. Or he may have become stuck on maintenance prescribing, the client being unable, or unwilling, to move away from a stabilising prescription of, for instance, methadone.

There are many other health and social care professionals that can be drawn into the integrated care pathway approach. Often criminal justice professionals can be involved: probation, youth offending teams, teams offering services in response to Drug Treatment and Testing Orders. Mark came into contact with drug services through his overdose, but it could have been following an arrest and a referral being made following contact with an arrest-referral worker, perhaps based in a police custody suite. Another point of access is following release from prison. The risk of overdose after a spell in prison is heightened as people will develop reduced tolerance. Where someone is highly likely to use substances on release, referral to local drug services can help minimise risk.

Finally, we must also acknowledge the important links with mental health services and the need for services to work with people who have what has been termed 'dual diagnosis' – co-morbidity of a substance and mental health problem. It seems to me that with more substance misusers tending towards polydrug use, with drugs becoming arguably stronger in their effect, and with drug use starting at a much earlier age, we can expect more people with complex health needs and at an earlier age. While the client, Mark, was not portrayed as having a mental health problem, many clients do: either the effect of the substance use, or a condition predating it that the client has sought to alleviate through substance use. In many areas 'dual diagnosis' services have been established. Other models involve stronger liaison links between generic substance misuse and mental health services. It is a challenging area and perhaps Models of Care can offer a clear framework for collaborative working with this client group, with substance misuse services providing specialist input for clients receiving treatment and support within mental health services. It will be vital for mental health treatment modalities to be in some way interfaced with the Models of

Care framework to ensure that this group of people receive appropriate and effective service provision.

We must also not forget young people. There will also need to be clear linkages with services for young people to ensure the smooth transition from young persons' to adult services, so that treatments and support may be continued with the minimum of disruption. The patterns of drug use of young people will provide the basis for the emphasis of future drug service provision. We are in many ways still learning what long-term effects single or polydrug use has on bodies and brains that are still developing. I have certainly experienced clients as adults whose emotional development has been arrested by heavy substance use during formative, teenage years. Drug services can surely expect to find themselves working with more complex situations, with greater numbers of people whose drug use has significantly impacted on their physical, emotional and mental health from a much earlier age.

Recently as well we see increasing emphasis on identifying and responding to the needs of the non-user(s) within, for instance, family systems where a substance-affected member is impacting on the system and the health and well-being of individuals. The scale of this problem is enormous; for instance, the reports indicate that there are 'between 250,000 and 350,000 children of problem drug users in the UK – about one for every problem drug user' (ACMD, 2003, p. 3). This is not to suggest that drug users are bad parents; we need to ensure that this assumption is not reinforced, remembering that each person is individual, as is their pattern and the effects of their drug using and associated behaviours. However, the report does make the point that 'parental problem drug use can and does cause serious harm to children at every age from conception to adulthood' (ACMD, 2003, p. 3).

The same report makes it clear that reducing the harm to children within problem drug-using family systems 'should become a main objective of policy and practice' (ACMD, 2003, p. 3). Collaborative treatment responses are therefore to be encouraged. We can also extend this concern beyond the needs of children adversely affected by drug use within family systems to other members of those families. Indeed, drug services are often called on to offer support to partners or parents of drug users. With this in mind it is heartening to observe that non-user support groups are being established, providing not only a welcome support for people so affected, but another group of informed people who can themselves inform service development and service provision.

Models of Care embraces a wide range of professions and professionals, and requires clear linkage with other, non-substance misuse specific services. Mark's story highlights some of the relationships and collaborative working that will be required. For some clients it will be more complex, for others less so. All must be catered for.

Is Models of Care an effective strategy for services to adopt to help clients with substance misuse problems? Time will tell. Perhaps, more than anything else, its effectiveness as a system will be governed by the quality and the transparency in the communication between services, the clarity of professional roles, a genuine evidence base (and one that also has scope for acknowledging the practice-based evidence that has developed within services in response to local needs), the level of collaborative working that is achieved and the degree to which the client is involved and owns the treatment packages that are formulated for him or her.

Will the treatment modalities be centred simply on the substance-using behaviours and effects, or will a more holistic perspective be established? Will multidisciplinary working and packages of treatment and care from various agencies support and enable the client to move on, or will they cause confusion, community institutionalisation, and possibly enhance fragmentation within the client's structure of self? Will services be 'substance-centred', 'patient-centred' or 'person-centred'?

What about client or 'user' involvement. I'm never too sure if 'user' is the best word – it narrows the description of the person and, in substance misuse services, not only equates to people as 'service users' but also 'drug users'. Yet one of the most important developments in recent years – and it continues to grow in strength and involvement – is the user group movement. Service users can be found not only running peer support groups, but taking a vocal and active part in the design, planning and implementation of treatment. Service users are participating in recruitment processes for staff in drug services; having a place at the table of drug reference groups and other service-specific groups, Drug Action Teams and other groups where strategies are developed and discussed.

Without doubt, Models of Care is forcing service providers and commissioners of services to sit down, evaluate local drug service provision and work towards ensuring effective services within their regions. It is producing the need to map out exactly what is being offered and by whom, to seek to ensure a range of treatment modalities is available, while avoiding unnecessary duplication. This is positive. It is bringing service providers together, with the hope of enhancing a collaborative culture. The 'bidding wars' between services, desperate to empire build and take over service provision from less entrepreneurial services, must surely become a thing of the past. But will it? And how smooth will the transitions be when clients are referred on, when care co-ordinators seek to draw together care pathways into an integrated package of care across agencies? Collaboration has to be the way forward – statutory and non-statutory agencies drawn together in a co-ordinated fashion with Drug Action Teams providing the necessary strategic overview to plan appropriate levels and types of service provision.

While it seems to me that Models of Care offers an opportunity for services to genuinely collaborate in such a way as to ensure that clients, wherever they live, are offered equity of access and service provision, it surely must offer more than this to be truly revolutionary – or should that be evolutionary? More than anything else, the establishing of the Models of Care framework and the system of integrated care pathways must *put the client at the heart of service provision*. I can think of no better emphasis to end this volume, offering, as it does, an experiential introduction to the application of Models of Care from a healthcare perspective.

References

- Advisory Council on the Misuse of Drugs (ACMD) (2003) *Hidden Harm: responding to the needs of children of problem drug users*. HMSO, London.

- Bryant-Jefferies R (2001) *Counselling the Person Beyond the Alcohol Problem*. Jessica Kingsley, London.

- Department of Health (2002) *Dual Diagnosis Good Practice Guide*. DoH, London.

- Health Advisory Service (1996) *Children and Young People: substance misuse services. The substance of young need*. HMSO, London.

- National Treatment Agency (NTA) (2002) *Models of Care for the Treatment of Drug Misusers: promoting quality, efficiency and effectiveness in drug misuse treatment services in England. Part 2: Full reference report*. National Treatment Agency for Substance Misuse, London.

- Skills for Health (2002) *Drugs and Alcohol National Occupational Standards (DANOS)*. Skills for Health, London.

- Substance Misuse Advisory Service (1999) *Commissioning Standards for Drug and Alcohol Treatment and Care*. Health Advisory Service, London.

- Velleman R (2001) *Counselling for Alcohol Problems*. Sage, London.

- www.skillsforhealth.org.uk: website of Skills for Health (formerly Healthworks UK).

Index

12-step programmes   12

abstinence   58, 130, 156
abuse   17, 118
acceptance (counselling)   99–101, 110
access to services   9–10, 155–6, 171
Acorn Community Drug and Alcohol
    Service   28
ACPC (Area Child Protection Committee)
    guidelines   21
acupuncture   128
aftercare   10, 11, 13, 157
AIDS (acquired immune deficiency
    syndrome)   11
alcohol
  care co-ordination   50, 55, 59, 87, 96–8,
      108
  counselling   99–101
  diaries   55, 97, 108
  and feelings   72–3, 75–6, 78–9, 84, 152
  and methadone   56, 61, 81, 96–101
  monitoring intake   127, 145
  and mother   87, 136, 138
  overdose   96–8, 136, 138
  prescribing clinics   50, 61, 150
  treatment services
    assessment   15–17
    care planning   18–21
    day programmes   89–90
    family therapy   160–1
    integrated care pathways   12–13
    monitoring   21–2
    Tiers 1–4 services   1, 8–12, 120
  triggers for drinking   43, 73, 74, 97
anger
  counselling   67, 70, 102, 124–5, 129,
      149
  day programmes   59

family background   50, 124–5
  at friends/peers   63
  mood diaries   52, 55
  at mother   48, 139
  sexual relationships   126–7
  using on top   48, 57
anxiety
  being clean   129
  care co-ordination   55, 56, 88, 131
  counselling   86, 103
  day programmes   59, 105, 107
  mood diary   55, 56
  moving out of area   88, 120, 131, 143–4
appointments   43–4, 47, 48, 118
appraisal   154
aromatherapy   128
arrests   10, 17, 165
assessment
  care co-ordination   58, 95, 119
  Level 1 (initial screening)   14, 27, 33
  Level 2 (triage)   15–16, 32–4
  Level 3 (comprehensive substance
      misuse)   16–18, 33–4, 43–4
  out of area   119, 120
  overview   2, 13–14, 23
  psychiatrist's perspective   154–5
attendance (non)   47, 48, 76, 112
auricular acupuncture   128
authenticity (counselling)   30, 34, 65, 99

belief systems   124, 160, 161
benefits (social security)   17, 106, 121
benzodiazepines (benzos)   56, 57, 59, 61, 98
Best Value frameworks   22
bidding wars   1, 120, 171
black populations   11, 22
blood-borne diseases   10, 17, 23, 169
boundary issues   36, 98, 154

brother, relationship with 68–70
buprenorphine (Subutex)
  day programmes 111, 117
  detoxification 61, 108, 130
  stabilisation 61, 118
  switching/reducing down 103–4,
    113–14, 117–18, 121–2, 124
  using on top 124, 150

cannabis 38, 51, 156
CARATS (Counselling, Assessment, Referral,
  Advice and Throughcare Services) 10
care co-ordination 8, 10–12, 18–21, 32–3,
  85
care co-ordinators
  care planning 19–21
  and counsellors 51, 54, 70, 135, 151
  inter-agency working 58, 90, 164, 171
  out of area 118–21, 131, 143
  psychiatrist's perspective 155–6
  role 44, 74, 94–5, 151, 160
  supervision 23–4, 98
  tiered treatment 11–12, 18, 32–3, 41
care pathways see also integrated care
  pathways
  care co-ordination 18–19, 33, 51, 58,
    171
  detoxification 168
  Models of Care 2, 7–8
  outreach workers 36
care planning 10, 18–19, 24, 155
care plans 11, 45–6, 58, 94, 153, 168–9
Care Programme Approach (CPA) 20, 156
CDATs see Community Drug and Alcohol
  Teams
change 82–5, 89–90, 124–5, 159–61,
  169
chasing (heroin) 55, 69
child protection 11, 14, 15, 21
childcare 9, 17
childhood experience 68–9, 73–4, 86–7,
  118
children 'at risk' 17, 43, 170
choice, and change 82, 85, 142, 161
choking 55, 96
clean works (needles) 30–2, 35, 37–8, 42,
  79, 97
'client-centred' treatment
  care co-ordination 19, 24
  day programmes 150

inter-agency working 120
  Models of Care 24, 154, 170–1
  overview iv, 2
clinical governance 22, 154, 157
clucking see withdrawal
cocaine 105, 112
cognitive-behavioural work 54, 74, 95,
  168
commissioning services 22, 171
Community Drug and Alcohol Service 66,
  70
Community Drug and Alcohol Teams
  (CDATs) 58
community support
  out of area 119, 128
  tiered treatment 8, 135
  work experience 168
  workers 51, 119, 141
co-morbidity 11, 17, 20, 23, 169
complementary therapies 23, 128–9
confidentiality
  attendance 77
  care co-ordination 21, 94
  counselling 65, 94, 122–4
  day programmes 106
  informal contact 41
consultants 156
coping skills 73, 84
counselling
  alcohol 99–101
  anger 49–51, 67, 102, 124–5, 129, 149
  anxiety 86, 103
  and care co-ordinators 54–5, 60, 74,
    94–6, 135, 151
  confidentiality 65, 94, 122–4
  empathy 99–103, 109–10, 122, 125
  feelings 72, 78, 81
  listening 66–7, 69, 70, 86
  Models of Care 2, 22, 155
  moving out of area 85, 114, 131–2
  non-attendance 47, 76
  outreach workers 30, 33
  Tier 3 services 10–11, 53
  work experience 130, 132, 136, 144
cousin, relationship with 64–5, 69–70
CPA see Care Programme Approach
criminal justice services 1, 9–10, 23–4,
  169
crisis intervention 12, 21, 137, 138
custody 9, 169

DANOS *see* Drug and Alcohol National
    Occupational Standards
DATs *see* Drug Action Teams
day programmes
    assessment 89–91
    care co-ordination 51, 57–8, 63, 83–4,
        107–8, 120
    group support 141–2, 145, 150
    life stories 105–6, 112, 128
    Models of Care 22, 160
    out of area 85, 120
    switching/reducing down 104–5, 108,
        111, 117
    tiered treatment 10–11, 47
de Bono, Edward 153
dealers
    availability of drugs 112
    distance from 30
    safety of drugs 28, 151
    seeing other users 61, 63, 82, 118
Department of Health iv, 20
dependency
    alcohol 17, 97
    drugs 16, 56, 151
    relationships 107, 110
'Dependency to Work' initiative 91
depressants 106
depression 17, 20, 56, 68, 72
designer drugs 1, 151
detoxification
    acupuncture 128
    anger 50
    buprenorphine (Subutex) 61, 104–5,
        108, 111, 113–14
    care plans 94
    day programmes 111, 150
    hospitals 28, 34, 41, 168
    tiered treatment 10, 11, 117
    young people 23
diaries
    alcohol 55, 97, 108
    mood 52, 55, 56, 59
diazepam 57
disability 17, 20, 47, 157
disappointment 72–5, 153
discharge from care 18, 38, 41, 43, 50,
    119
disengagement from services 13, 15, 17, 19
doctors 30 *see also* GPs
domestic violence 17

dope 106
'double-scripting' 45
drop-in facilities 10, 29, 37, 44, 47
drop-out rates iv, 19, 128, 155
Drug Action Teams (DATs) iv, 1, 71–2, 171
Drug and Alcohol National Occupational
    Standards (DANOS) 14, 21
drug misuse
    guilt 53–4
    memories of 31–2, 62–4, 82–3, 129
    professionals' experience 100
drug services
    accommodation 113
    assessment 13–18
    care planning/co-ordination 18–21
    day programmes 89, 106, 112
    family therapist's perspective 159–61
    integrated care pathways 12–13
    inter-agency working 24, 120
    monitoring 21–2
    overview iv, 1–3, 7–8, 167–71
    psychiatrist's perspective 153–7
    tiered treatment 8–12
    treatment modalities 22–3
    work experience 130
Drug Treatment and Testing Orders
    (DTTOs) 11, 12, 20, 157, 169
dual diagnosis
    integrated care pathways 169
    Models of Care 8, 12, 20, 23
    psychiatrist's perspective 154, 156

ECPA (Enhanced Care Programme Approach)
    20
emergency care 15, 16
emotions *see* feelings
empathy (counselling) 99–103, 109–10,
    122, 125
employment *see* work experience
endings, processing 131, 145
Enhanced Care Co-ordination 20
Enhanced Care Programme Approach
    (ECPA) 20
ethnic background 19, 20
evidence base 154, 170–1

faith-based programmes 12
family issues
    assessment 17, 23, 44
    care co-ordination 73–4, 88

counselling 68–9, 99, 124–5
day programmes 91, 142
family therapy 10–11, 159–61, 168
GP's knowledge 155
non-users 170
outreach workers 33, 38
substitute family 130, 142
tiered treatment 10–11
father, relationship with 50, 68–9, 125
feelings
   alcohol 72, 78–9, 84, 108
   care co-ordination 75, 107–8
   counselling 66, 86–7, 102–4, 114, 129, 136
   day programmes 90, 112, 141–2
   methadone 49–50, 84, 102
   non-attendance 76
   reducing down 104, 107, 114, 129
   stabilisation 81
   using on top 78–9
fixes, organising 36, 48, 97
forensic services 12
friends 62–4, 72, 82, 118–19, 131
frustration 73–5, 103, 113, 151
funding
   assessment 18, 120
   complementary therapies 128
   drug treatment 7, 37, 70
   moving out of area 118, 120
   psychiatrist's perspective 155, 157

gear 28 *see also* heroin
gender issues 19–21, 125
genito-urinary medicine 12
GPs
   assessment 44–5
   liaison out of area 118–19, 131–2
   psychiatrist's perspective 155–6
   stabilisation 169
group work
   day programmes 51, 91, 105–6, 113, 117, 141–2
   family therapy 160, 170
   outreach workers 33
   support 51, 113, 138, 170
   user involvement 171
guilt 53

habit 83, 84, 151
harm minimisation
   confidentiality 122–3
   injecting users 29–31, 64
   Models of Care 9, 15
   outreach workers 30–1, 151
   supervised consumption 77–8, 130
   young people 23, 170
health needs 9, 94–5, 157, 169
helplines 45, 108
hepatitis B/C 9, 12, 27, 29, 35, 169
heroin (gear/smack)
   and alcohol 55, 90, 96
   assessment 28, 34, 35
   and buprenorphine (Subutex) 61
   counselling 69, 104
   and feelings 31–2, 49–50, 55, 62–4, 81, 108
   outreach workers 31, 35
   overdose 28, 35
   using on top 48–9, 56–7
HIV (human immunodeficiency virus) 11, 12, 27, 29, 169
holding onto clients 15, 18, 120
'holding' doses 42, 45, 46, 56
holistic treatment 18, 24, 129, 156, 171
homelessness 9, 11
hospitals
   discharge from care 38, 50
   inter-agency working 120, 155
   ward assessment 27–30, 33–4, 38, 150
hostels 9
housing 8–9, 11, 17, 168

ICPs *see* integrated care pathways
implementation targets 7–8, 167
informal support 29, 31–3, 36, 38, 47, 151
injecting users
   assessment 28–9, 34, 44, 151
   buprenorphine (Subutex) 104, 111
   clean works 30–2, 35, 37–8, 42, 79, 97
   crushed tablets 104, 111
   harm minimisation 30–1, 37, 64
   infections 31, 37, 97, 169
   memories of drug use 54–5, 62–3
   Models of Care 8, 10
   outreach workers 30–1, 33, 37
inpatient treatment 11–12, 22, 46, 156, 168

integrated care pathways (ICPs)
  care co-ordinators   24, 33, 95
  inter-agency working   120, 169–70
  Models of Care   8, 12–13, 24, 154, 171
intensive care   27, 138
inter-agency working   23, 58, 90–1, 120,
  138, 170–1
irritation   73–5, 98, 107–8

jacking up   30, 62, 63, 68
junkies   54, 97

leaflets   31, 37–8, 52, 105, 120–1, 160
Level 1 assessment (initial screening)   14,
  27, 33
Level 2 assessment (triage)   14–16, 27, 29,
  32–3, 38
Level 3 assessment (comprehensive substance
  misuse)   16–18, 27, 33, 37, 41
liaison out of area   34, 117–21, 128, 145
life lines   82–5, 87, 89, 91, 95–8, 152
life stories   118
listening (in counselling)   66–7, 69, 70, 86
liver disorders   12, 17, 139
local services, variation in   64–5, 85, 128,
  171
losses   129, 131

maintenance programmes
  buprenorphine (Subutex)   104, 111
  day programmes   58–9, 106, 111
  liaison out of area   119
  methadone   10, 59, 169
  Tier 3 services   10–11
memories of drug use   62–4, 82–3, 113,
  129
mental health
  assessment   16–18, 33, 37, 44
  care co-ordination   20, 47, 94–5
  dual diagnosis   8, 20, 23, 154, 156,
    169
  Mental Health Act   20
  tiered treatment   11–12
meta-studies (family therapy)   160
methadone
  and alcohol   96–9, 101
  and benzodiazepines   56–7
  and buprenorphine (Subutex)   61, 103,
    111, 113, 121

  care co-ordination   49–50, 55, 84, 96–8,
    108, 113
  counselling   66, 99, 101–4
  day programmes   59, 90, 105
  and feelings   49–50, 55, 73, 78–9, 84, 108
  maintenance programmes   10, 32, 41,
    59, 111, 169
  moving out of area   64–5, 71, 85
  non-attendance   76–7
  prescribing   42, 44–6, 48–50, 61, 81
  switching/reducing down   90–1, 114,
    122–4
  using on top   48–9, 56–7, 80, 122–4,
    149–50
  withdrawal   114, 121
Milan approaches (family therapy)   161
minority ethnic populations   11, 22
mirroring language   126
mobile phones   38, 41, 46, 150
Models of Care
  care planning/co-ordination   18–21, 32,
    54, 168
  family therapist's perspective   159–61
  implementation   7–8, 153, 168
  integrated care pathways   12–13
  inter-agency working   90, 120, 138, 170
  Level 1 assessment (initial screening)
    13–14
  Level 2 assessment (triage)   13, 15–16
  Level 3 assessment (comprehensive
    substance misuse)   14, 16–18
  monitoring   21–2
  overview   iv, 1–3, 7–8, 167–71
  psychiatrist's perspective   153–7, 167
  Tier 1 services   8–9
  Tier 2 services   9–10
  Tier 3 services   10–11
  Tier 4 services   11–12
  treatment modalities   22–3
monitoring   21–2, 95, 113–14, 127
mood monitoring
  care co-ordination   52–3, 55–6, 59,
    97, 145
  day programmes   112
  mood diaries   52, 55–6, 59
mother, relationship with
  care co-ordination   53–4, 74–5, 87–9,
    151
  client's drug use   43, 48, 50, 54

mother, relationship with (*continued*)
  counselling   66, 68–9, 86–9, 99, 125, 149
  family therapy   159–61, 168
  improvement in   87, 144–5, 152
  mother's drug use   41, 44, 54, 74
  mother's overdose   44, 136–40, 149, 159
  reaction to moving away   87–9, 130–1, 142–3
motivational work   9–10, 36, 50, 56, 95, 120
moving out of area
  life lines   85, 91
  local drug services   3, 64–5, 70, 114, 131–2
  mother's reaction   87–9, 130–1, 142–3
multidisciplinary working   18, 156, 171

Narcotics Anonymous (NA)   59, 119
narrative approaches (family therapy)   161
National Service Frameworks   iv, 156
National Treatment Agency on Substance Misuse (NTA)   iv, 1, 7–8, 22
needles
  clean works   30–2, 35, 37–8, 42, 79, 97
  needle exchange   9, 10, 22, 38, 41–3
  outreach work   30, 35, 37, 41, 137
NHS   22, 70, 118
non-users (family therapy)   170
NTA *see* National Treatment Agency on Substance Misuse
nurse consultant, reflections   163–5
nurses   27, 30, 34, 50, 94, 155

occupational therapy   168
open access treatment   2, 9–10
openness (in counselling)   65, 68, 110, 118
opiates   21, 33, 56, 112
opioids   9, 61
outreach workers
  assessment   32–8, 154
  crisis intervention   137–41
  harm minimisation   29–31, 34–7
  inter-agency working   47, 120
  reducing down   127, 129
  Tier 2 services   10, 23, 29–30, 117, 135
  view of client   150–1
overdose
  assessment   14–15, 17, 28, 34–5, 44
  buprenorphine (Subutex)   61

day programmes   89, 112, 117
harm minimisation   38, 64, 77, 80
Models of Care   10, 23, 169–70
of mother   44, 136–40, 149, 159
using on top   42, 45, 79–80, 130

paracetamol   136, 138
parasuicide   14
parenting   9, 22, 68–9, 170
partners   17, 170
'person-centred' treatment   22, 86, 171
pharmacies   9–10, 45, 64, 70–1
police   9, 157, 169
polydrug use   21, 169
'postcode lottery'   iv
post-structural stance (family therapy)   160
pregnancy   9, 11, 17
prescribing clinics
  local drug services   71, 85, 118–19, 157
  stabilisation   94, 169
  substitute prescribing   16, 33, 42, 154, 156
  Tier 3 services   42–6, 135
  using on top   130, 149–50
primary healthcare   9, 118, 119, 169
prisons   8, 10, 12, 17, 169
probation services   9, 17, 20, 169
psychiatric problems   11, 23
psychiatrist's perspective, Models of Care   153–7
psychological problems   17, 151, 168
psychotherapy   10, 160
psychotic users   156

QuADS standards (Quality in Alcohol and Drug Services)   22
questionnaires   106, 145
'quick fixes'   36, 49, 84–5, 115

rape   118
reducing down
  buprenorphine (Subutex)   111, 114, 118, 127, 129
  day programmes   90, 106, 111
  methadone   90–1, 94, 103–4
rehabilitation services   10–12, 22, 36, 43, 50, 168
relapse prevention
  care co-ordinators   62–3, 74
  group work   89, 135

outreach work 33, 141
shared care 118
relationships *see also* mother, relationship
    with
brother 68–70
cousin 64–5, 69–70
day programmes 90, 128
dependency 106–7, 110
family therapy 159–61, 168
father 50, 68–9, 125
sexual relations 106, 121, 123, 126–8,
    152
stepfather 68–9, 75, 99, 124–5
relaxation 59, 65, 67, 72, 113, 128
residential services 8, 10–12, 223, 36, 168
respect (in counselling) 31, 34, 99
respiratory failure 55, 96
risk assessment 14–16, 19–20, 41, 151,
    154

sadness 129, 139, 149
schizophrenia 20
school problems 50, 69, 74, 91
scoring
avoiding feelings 72, 78–9, 97
definition 38
life lines 82–3
money for 42, 47–9
SCPA *see* Standard Care Programme
    Approach
scripts (family therapy) 161
scripts (methadone) 41 *see also* methadone
second opinions 109
sedation 46, 96
self-belief 124
self-disclosing 100
self-harm 14–17, 122–3
self-help groups 23
service users 2, 20–2, 24, 171
'service-centred' treatment iv, 120
sexual abuse 118
sexual relations 106, 121, 123, 126–8, 152
sexuality 19, 20
shame 54
shared care 9, 11, 118–19
sharing works 97 *see also* clean works
shoplifting 42
sickness benefit 106
silence (in counselling) 31, 66, 99–100,
    142

skunk 156
smack 28, 31, 54–5, 63, 73 *see also* heroin
smoking
heroin 54, 63
tobacco 127
social services 11, 24, 125
social work 9, 18, 33, 51, 120, 168
solution-focused approach (family
    therapy) 161
speed (amphetamine) 112
stabilisation
buprenorphine (Subutex) 61, 114
methadone 48, 80–1, 90–1, 93, 97, 169
Models of Care 11, 18, 155
prescribing clinics 48, 61, 80–1, 93
shared care 118
Standard Care Co-ordination 20
Standard Care Programme Approach
    (SCPA) 20
stealing 47, 48, 63, 121
stepfather, relationship with 68–9, 75, 99,
    124–5
stimulants 11, 21, 22, 106
stress 81, 99, 151
substance misuse *see also* drug misuse; drug
    services
assessment 34
avoiding feelings 31–2, 50, 72–3
day programmes 90, 105, 112
overview 1–3, 167–71
professionals' experience 100
shared care 118–19
tobacco 127
'substance-centred' treatment 171
substitute prescribing 16, 33, 42, 154,
    156
Subutex *see* buprenorphine
suicide 14, 15, 44, 88
supervised consumption
harm minimisation 42, 46, 77, 130
moving out of area 65, 70–1, 85
prescribing clinics 45–6, 52, 93
supervision
for care co-ordinators 23, 98
for counsellors 101, 125
outreach workers 36
psychiatrist's perspective 154
support services
care co-ordinators 51, 160
moving out of area 85, 87, 89, 114, 119

support services (*continued*)
  Narcotics Anonymous   59, 119
  support groups   37, 47
  user groups   171
suppressant effect, methadone   55, 56, 97
swearing   126, 154
syringes   30, 35

tablets, injecting   104, 111
teenagers *see* young people
therapeutic counselling *see* counselling
therapeutic relationship   70, 100
therapists   94, 95, 100 *see also* counselling
threatening behaviour   15, 122–3
tiered treatment
  assessment   13–16
  overview   2, 7
  psychiatrist's perspective   156
  Tier 1 services
    hepatitis B/C   27, 35
    hospital ward assessment   27–8, 33, 35
    Models of Care   8–10, 13
    training   52, 120
  Tier 2 services
    day programmes   53, 61, 77, 93, 117, 135
    drug services   41, 45, 47
    liaison out of area   117, 120
    Models of Care   8–10, 16
    outreach work   27–9, 34, 36, 120, 135
    professionals' drug use   100
  Tier 3 services
    assessment   16–18, 27, 29, 34
    care co-ordination   32, 47, 117–18, 135, 160
    liaison out of area   117, 118, 120
    methadone maintenance   52–3, 61, 77, 93, 169
    Models of Care   2, 8, 10–11
    prescribing clinics   41, 42, 52, 135
    therapeutic counselling   52–3, 61, 77, 93, 117–18, 135
  Tier 4 services   10–12, 16, 155
  young people   23
time, use of   47, 51–2, 57–8, 105, 157
tiredness
  care co-ordination   75, 96
  counselling   68, 100, 102–3, 125
  day programmes   106

tobacco   127
tolerance testing   155, 169
training
  assessment   2, 16, 23, 120
  counselling   100, 132, 144
  psychiatrist's perspective   154, 157
  Tier 1 services   9, 51–2, 120
tranquillisers   56, 81
trans-generational framework (family therapy)   161
trauma   17, 74
treatment modalities   22, 33–4, 90–1, 163, 167–8, 169–71
'treatment-centred' approach   150
triage assessment   10, 15–16, 18, 32, 154
triggers
  for drinking   73, 74, 97
  relationships   111
  for using   62, 74
trips (drug effect)   106
trust
  counselling   86, 126
  day programmes   106, 117
  family therapy   160
  outreach workers   31
  using on top   79–80, 93, 127

unemployment   106
urine tests
  prescribing clinics   42–3, 45, 53, 57, 61, 93
  using on top   42, 45, 55–7, 93
used needles   37, 137
user groups   23, 128, 171
using on top
  care co-ordination   55, 151
  confidentiality   122–3
  prescribing clinics   42, 45–6, 61, 80, 130, 149–50
  urine tests   42, 45, 55–7, 93
  using off the streets   33, 48, 78

vaccinations   9, 29, 35
veins   12, 30–1, 34
violence   15, 17, 124–5
vocational training   51–2, 56
vodka   136, 138
vomiting   55, 96

warmth (in counselling)   99, 100, 110
withdrawal (clucking)
    assessment   16, 44
    buprenorphine (Subutex)   104–5, 114,
        121
    care co-ordination   50, 55, 64, 74
    heroin   44, 55, 64
    methadone   50, 77, 114
    mother's drug use   74
    prescribing clinics   44, 46

women drug misusers   11, 12, 22
work experience
    assessment   17
    counselling   130, 132, 136, 144
    day programmes   106
    returning to work   73, 91, 121, 130,
        151–2, 168
    vocational training   51–2, 56

young people   11–12, 22–3, 170